Inspecting the Newborn Baby's Eyes

ATLASES OF CHILDHOOD SERIES

Inspecting the Newborn Baby's Eyes

Neil O'Doherty, MD, FRCP, DCH

Associate Professor of Paediatrics
University College, Dublin

Consultant Paediatrician
The Children's Hospital
Temple Street, Dublin

MTP PRESS LIMITED
a member of the KLUWER ACADEMIC PUBLISHERS GROUP
LANCASTER / BOSTON / THE HAGUE / DORDRECHT

Published in the UK and Europe by
MTP Press Limited
Falcon House
Lancaster, England

British Library Cataloguing in Publication Data

O'Doherty, Neil
   Inspecting the newborn baby's eyes
   (Atlases of childhood series)
   1. Infants (Newborn)—Diseases—
   Diagnosis   2. Pediatric ophthalmology—
   Diagnosis
   I. Title   II. Series
   618.92′0977   RJ296

   ISBN-13: 978-94-010-8335-5   e-ISBN-13: 978-94-009-4137-3
   DOI: 10.1007/978-94-009-4137-3

Published in the USA by
MTP Press
A division of Kluwer Boston Inc
190 Old Derby Street
Hingham, MA 02043, USA

Typeset by Blackpool Typesetting Services Ltd., Blackpool
Colour origination by Laserscan Studios, Manchester
Printed by Cradely Print plc, Warley, W. Midlands
Bound by Butler and Tanner, Ltd., Frome and London

CONTENTS

ACKNOWLEDGEMENTS

Most of the photographs in Part I and many in Part II were obtained with the co-operation of the Department of Medical Photography, West Middlesex Hospital.

Guy's Hospital Medical School kindly permitted the use of material realized there by the author.

My colleagues generously complemented my own resources whenever possible. Because of their specialized interests some were especially prolific:

Mr Roger Bowell

Dr S. F. Cahalane FRCPath

Dr L. V. Deverajan (Kuwait)

Dr Niall O'Brien (National Maternity Hospital)

Mr Seamus O'Riain

Other contributors were:

Dr John Cosgrove

Dr Sylvia Dockeray

Dr Desmond Duff

Mr Ray Fitzgerald

Professor Denis Gill

Dr Winifred Gorman

Dr Elizabeth Griffin

Dr R. J. Hay

Dr Mary Kent

Dr Mary King

Dr Susan McManus (who kindly advised on the content and presentation of Appendix III)

Dr Tom Matthews

Dr J. N. Montgomery

Dr Eileen Naughten

Mr Hugh O'Donoghue

Professor N. V. O'Donohoe

Mr B. P. Prendiville

Dr Edward Tempany

The two slides of bilateral retinoblastoma (8A, 8B) are included by kind permission of *Modern Medicine of Ireland*.

PART I

ROUTINE UNIVERSAL OBSERVATIONS, BACKGROUND, TECHNIQUES AND FINDINGS

INTRODUCTION

It might on first impression seem excessive to devote even a modest volume just to a single sector of one system over the course of a few days. Justification depends on the fact that routine inspection of the eyes in current neonatal practice is embarrassingly unrewarding, yet easily capable of major improvement. Up to the present, little time seems to have been devoted to teaching the baby's physiological responses, yet nowhere is there more truth in the paediatric precept that success is founded in a thorough knowledge of the range of normal. If the eyes happened to be well open the aims of inspection, when expressed, may for instance have been pupil size, shape and reaction to light, cataract or coloboma. Such objections are unrealistic, relatively unrewarding and almost unachievable; for instance, to take but one item, coloboma 'prevalence figures are not available' (*Survey of Ophthalmology*, 1981) ... *res ipsa loquitur*.

The book has four main objectives.

(1) To portray the baby's relevant physiology and the primitive automatic responses that ensure full eye opening and maximum display. It is intended as learning aid and teaching manual for the junior doctor and his tutor, respectively. Points of technique are emphasized and possible pitfalls indicated.

(2) To show the items that constitute the *irreducible minimum* observable in every baby, the normal and pathological are portrayed.

(3) Beyond these basic items every other finding is a bonus discovered only occasionally but not so rare that every junior would not see at least several during his term. The rarities are rarely trivial, some are vitally urgent.

   When the unusual is in the offing it is the doctor well grounded in the normal who will do better: 'In the fields of observation chance favours only the mind that is prepared' (Pasteur, lecture).

(4) Here the physician's role is to direct the photographer; the camera's advantage as *privileged observer* is well shown, especially in magnifying close-up detail or catching frozen movement.

LEARNING FROM EXPERIENCE

Always listen to the mother, she is usually right.
(Mary Sheridan)

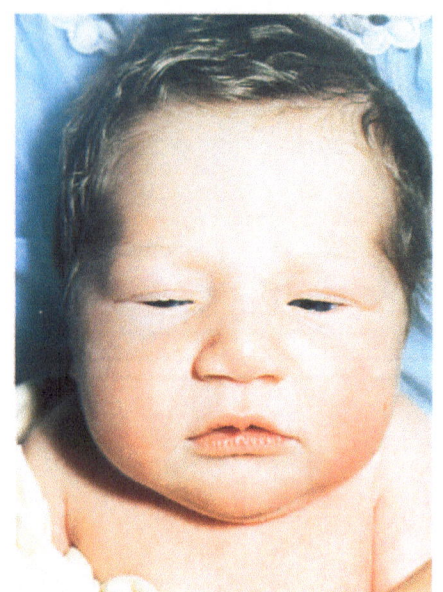

1 Best manoeuvre: doll's eye reflex

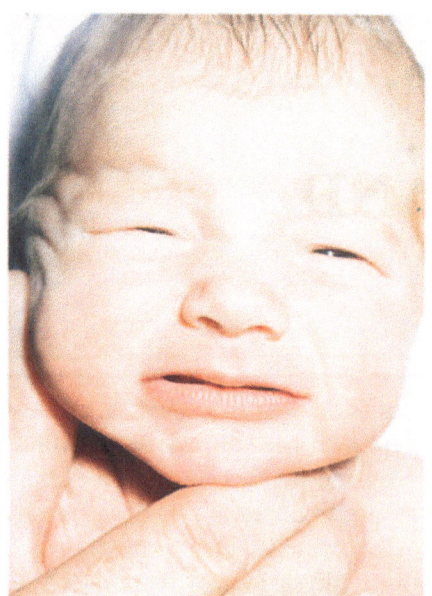

2 Best manoeuvre: auditory quietening response

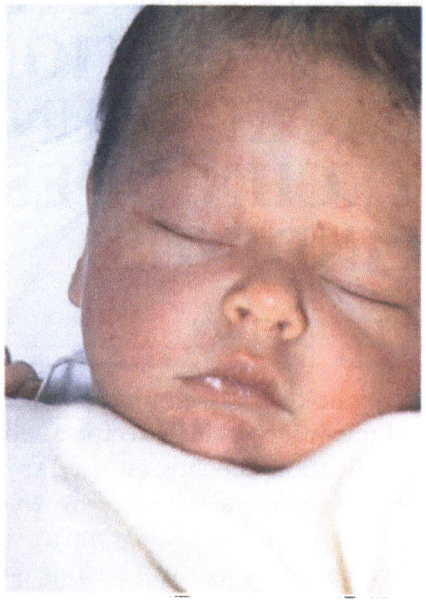

3 Best manoeuvre: let baby wake up

The primary care doctor must have the skill to make the baby display maximum eye-opening and then move the eyes about, thanks to some primitive reflexes. There is an irreducible minimum that should always be seen; this is usually functional and there is always the possible bonus of detecting something additional, generally of a structural nature.

Some faults are inevitable in any routine examination extensively applied and the commonest mistake is that the circumstances are allowed to militate against success when it is actually quite easy for the clinician to turn things to his advantage. For example, pitfalls as simple and as common as mild periorbital oedema [1] or a slight grizzly baby [2] would seriously impair *anybody's* chances unless he knew the simple measure to overcome the problem. Where the eyes are not opened satisfactorily, the commonest simple miss is subconjunctival haemorrhage; the associated tell-tale external marks of trauma, mechanical purpura [3], forceps mark [4] or black eye [5] should not be disregarded.

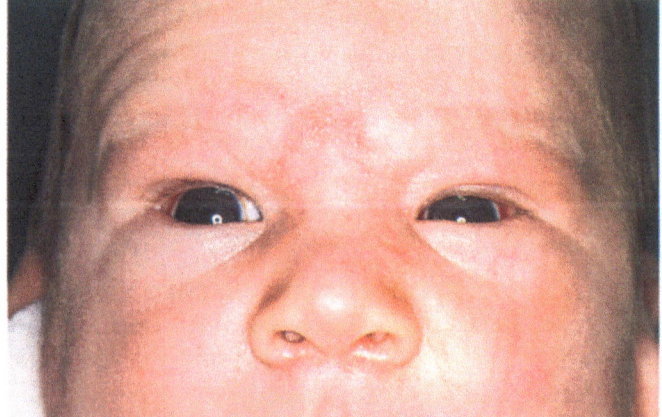

4 Haemorrhage at typical site close to iris . . .

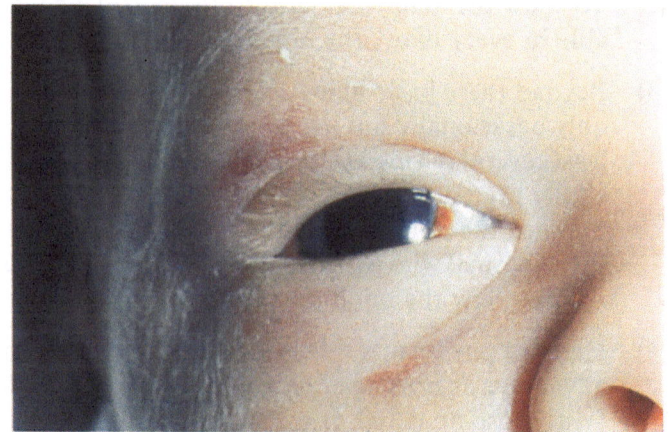

5 Red colour retained by diffusion of oxygen

8 INSPECTING THE NEWBORN BABY'S EYES

Leukokoria (white pupil) is the big omission, even cataract has been missed [6]; this mother says she told the nursery staff, family doctor and clinic doctor before she was referred to the paediatrician, for reassurance. In another case [7] bilateral cataract with jerky eye movements in a child with Down's syndrome went unremarked until she was 2 years old; since one cannot say if these were congenital, the facts serve only to show how something may be overlooked (even) in a 2-year-old *at risk*. Other possible causes of leukokoria are retrolental fibroplasia [8], retinoblastoma [8A, 8B, 9] and pseudoglioma. Early diagnosis means a better outcome in many regards, including willingness to accept aids such as glasses and prostheses [10].

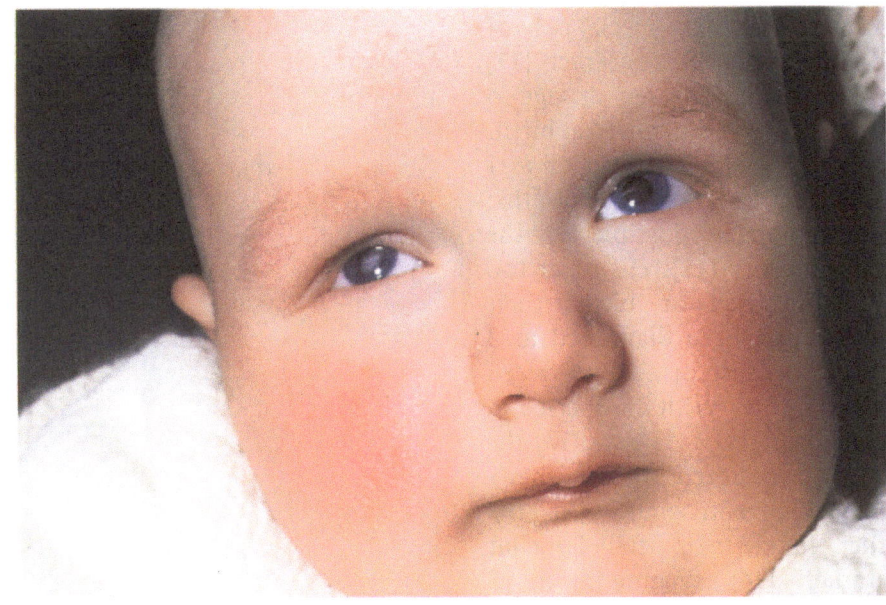

6 Probably squint in nursery as well

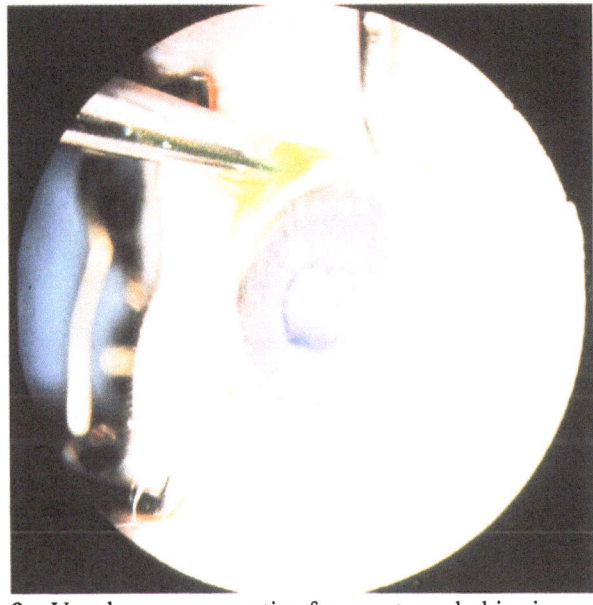

8 Usual nursery practice for pre-term babies is formal ophthalmoscopy*

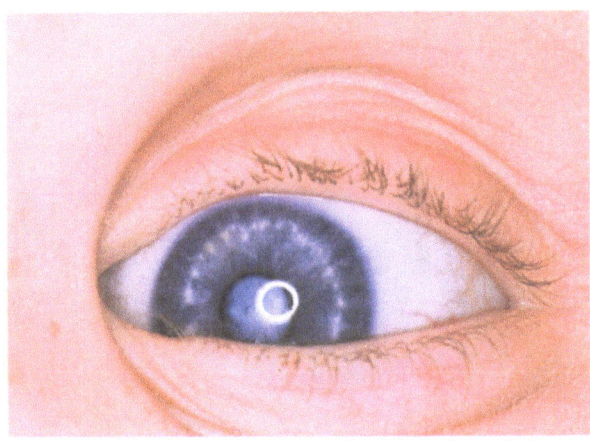

7 Brushfield spots in 10% of population, fade with age

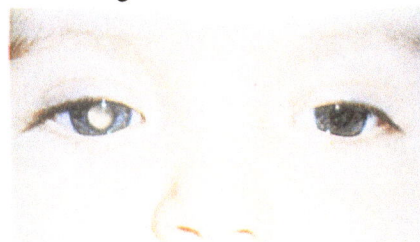

8A Leukocoria from retinoblastoma

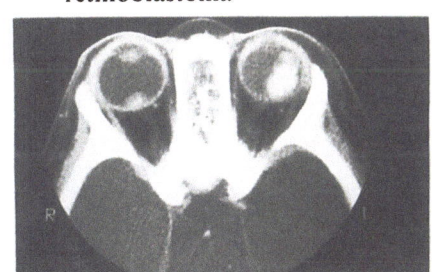

8B CT scan shows primary tumour and either metastasis or multifocal growth in second eye.

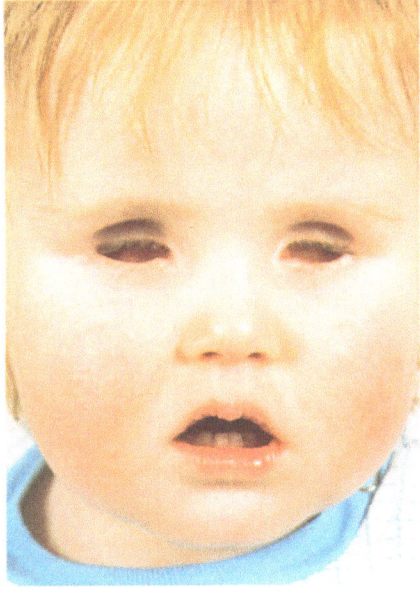

9 Bilateral enucleation in infancy . . .

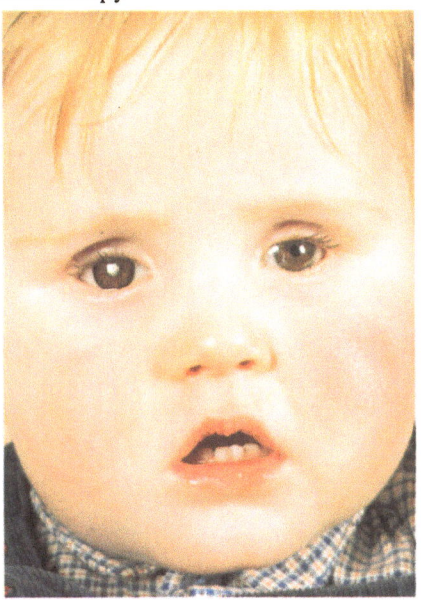

10 Prostheses readily accepted

*'La Gatta frettolosa fa i figli ciechi'
'The impatient cat begets blind kittens' (Italian proverb)

9

There was a very special case of dominant inherited cataract [11] who accepted glasses at age 4 months: he was diagnosed at birth, had the first side operated on at 1 month and the other at 3 months; this was made possible by the family history [12]. His sister too was diagnosed at birth; their mother had been diagnosed at 3 months because of a query raised by her father. With another child given glasses at 1½ years [13] the situation required that mother's vigilant inventiveness. On the other hand, a partial lamellar cataract [14] diagnosed at 2 months needed only to be kept under review until the optimum time for surgery arrived, at 20 months in this case.

Coloboma [15] is, for instance another blatant anomaly that continues to be missed in the nursery, simply for the want of a good look with the eyes properly opened. Possible masking [16] in its usual six o'clock position is only a partial feeble excuse [see also 191, 192]. In another instance [17] the arresting lip deformity of trisomy-13 may overshadow the bilateral medial coloboma notches at the four o'clock and eight o'clock position.

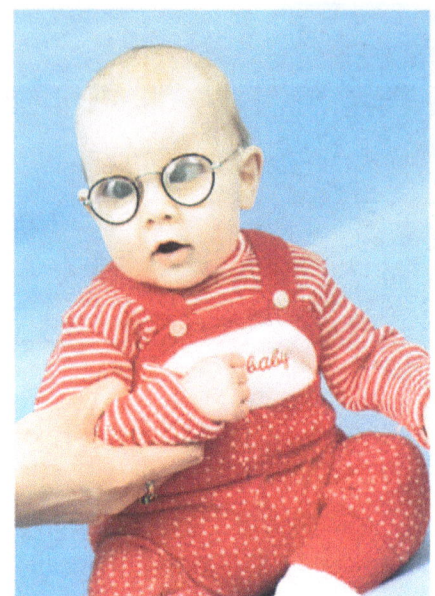

11 Spectacles readily accepted

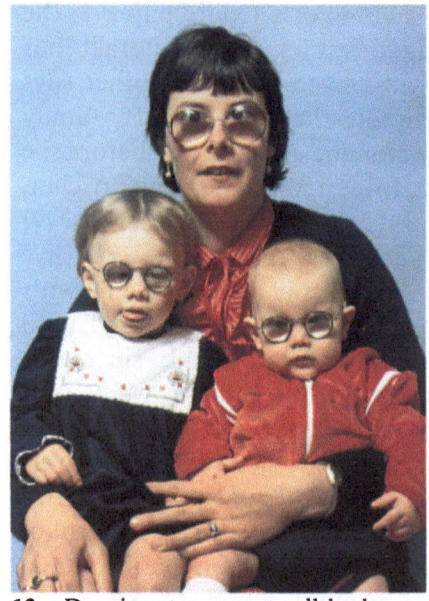

12 Dominant cataract: all had spectacles in first year

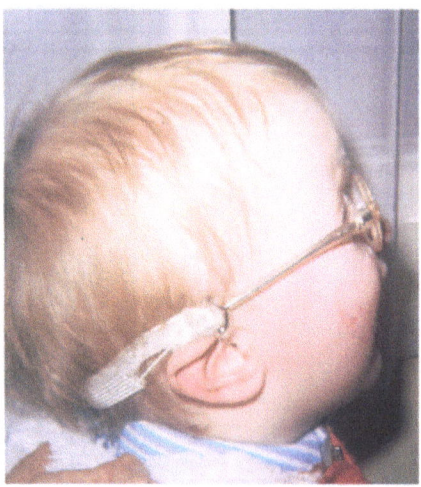

13 After infancy, spectacles are worn less readily

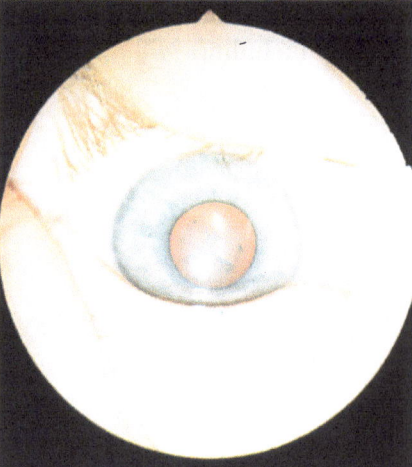

14

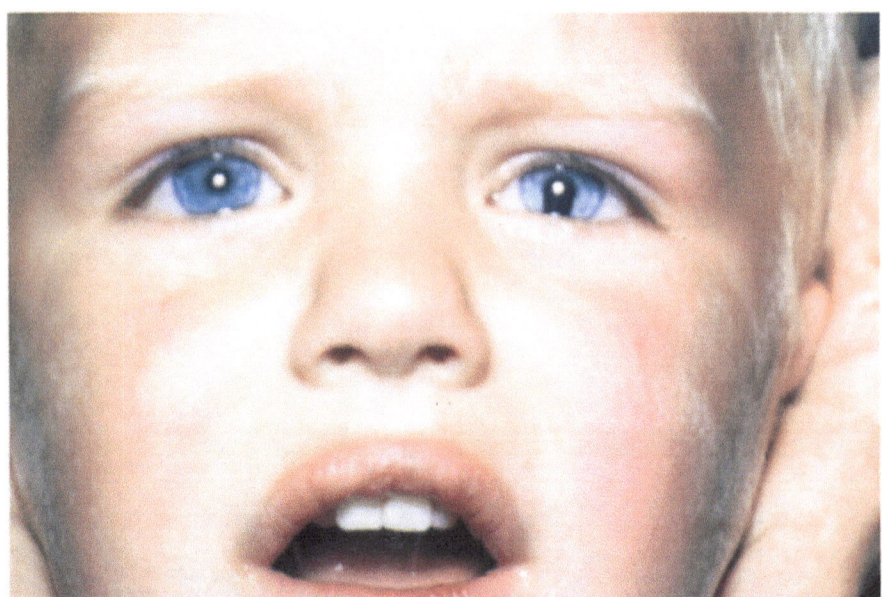

15 'Keyhole' iris

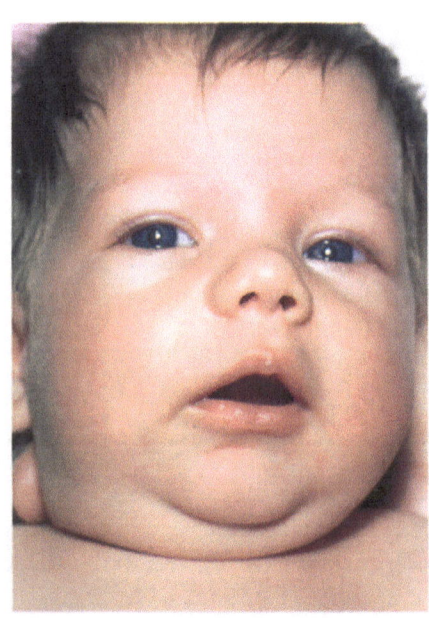

16 Left lid covers lower iris, thus concealing cataract

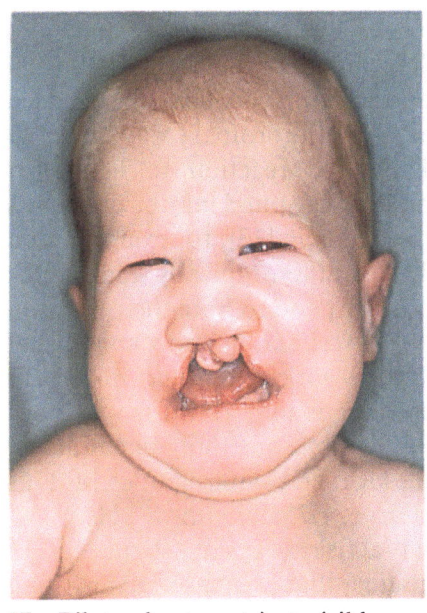

17 Bilateral cataract just visible

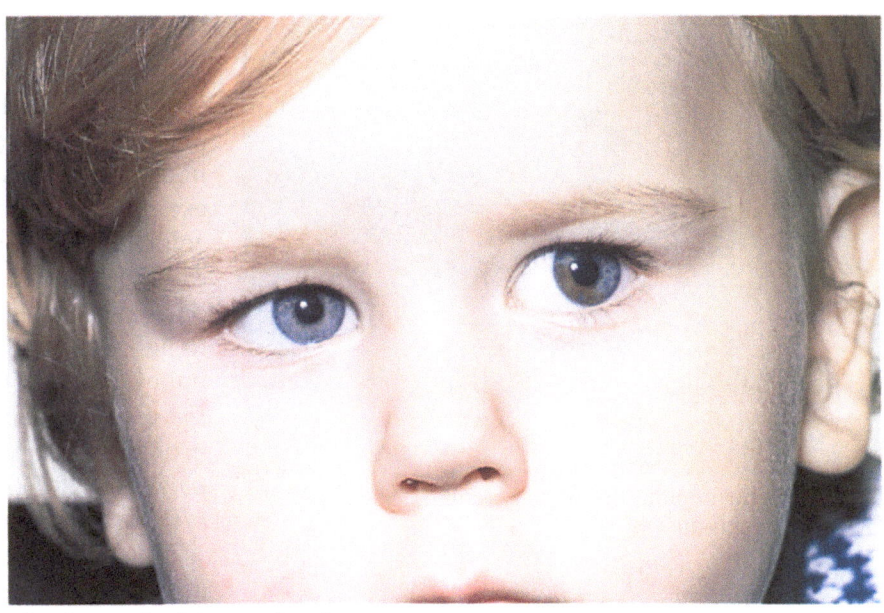

18 Recognized by mother in nursery

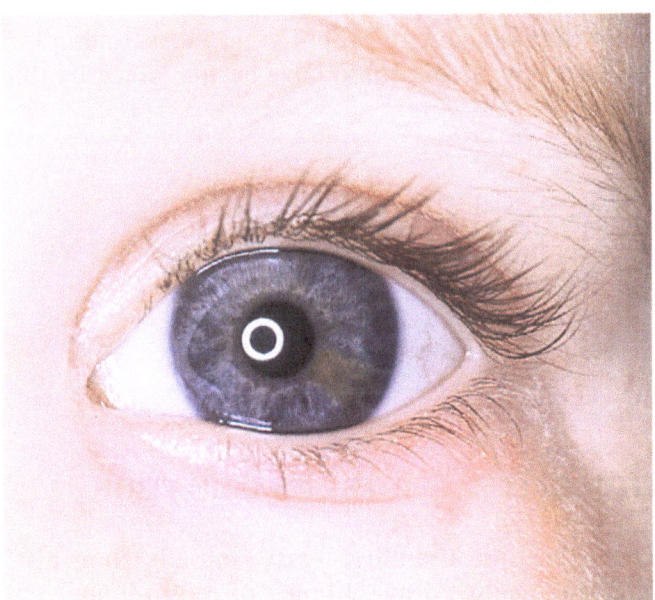

19

We can learn from the mother, she is an incomparable observer, always with the baby in his waking periods, she fixes him at the loving distance and searches his eyes continually, indeed their very *rapport* is a stimulus to wide eye opening. She always sees a subconjunctival haemorrhage and rarely misses the least little defect [18, 19]. One doctor's wife saw something that could not be confirmed; it was 6 months before she was vindicated when the ophthalmologist saw with a narrow beam [20] that there was a dot cataract in the six o'clock position. Another mother saw the eyes 'shimmering' which at first might suggest the possibility of some rarity such as cystinosis [21] but it turned out that the baby had rotatory nystagmus; this amateur description of the deft quick hairspring movement was very good indeed [**see also 175, 283–285**].

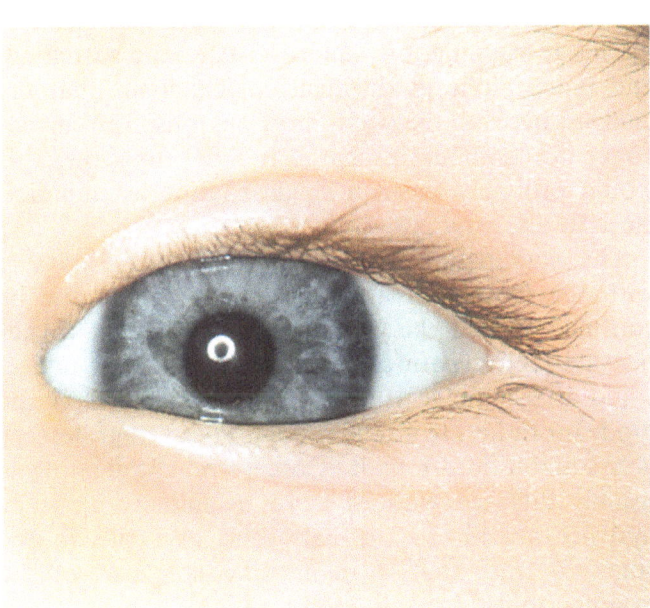

20 Tiny spicules at 6 o'clock

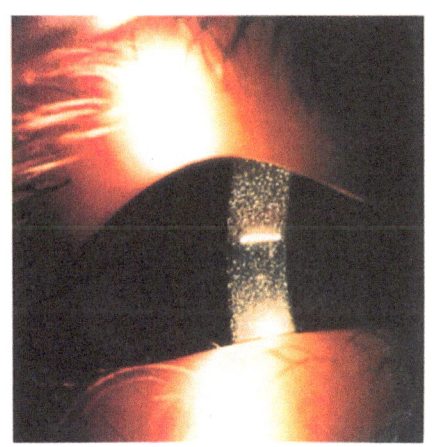

21

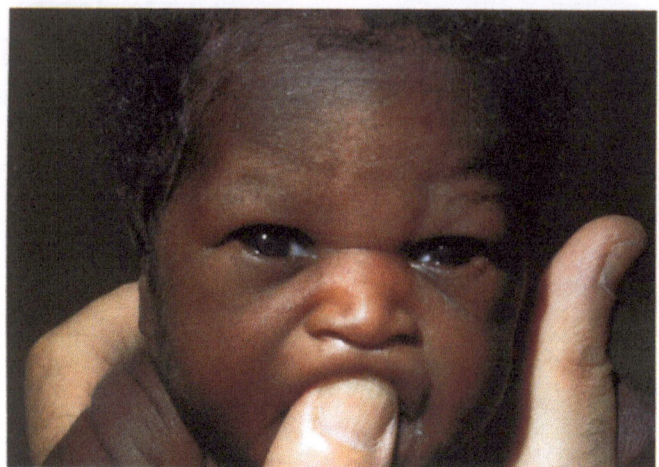

22 Rich brown colour seems to be common in non-Caucasians

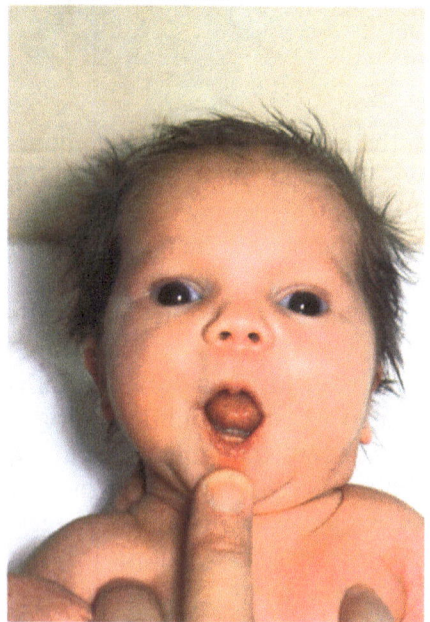

23 Typical 'wet' look

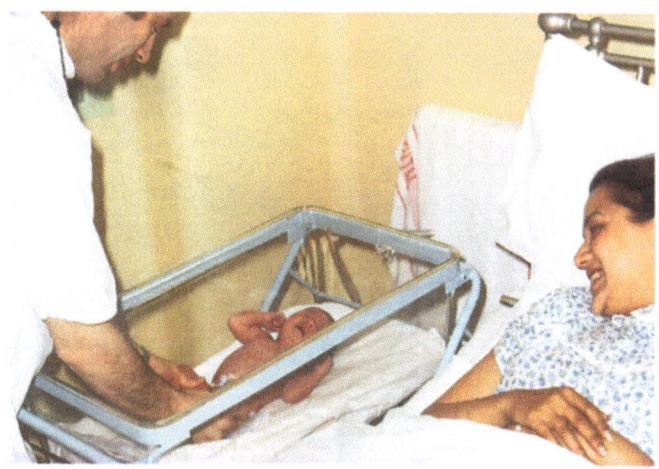

24 Nurses' eye view

The most important thing for the junior doctor to appreciate from the outset is that the hallowed approach of adult neurology has very little place indeed in the nursery; we cannot in the ordinary way expect to note pupil size, shape and reaction to light, for example. The invisibility of the pupil may be due to iris coloration [22] or reflected light [23], for example, and even with a good sighting of these typically small pupils one would have to be very good to note their reaction to light below the blink threshold, not only consensual but even direct. In routine work, *it is simply not worth the effort:* when pupil size is important, it will in all probability be semaphored by something like brachial palsy [see 204] (small, Horner's syndrome) or Möbius syndrome [see 162] (large, III oculomotor palsy).

Finally it is a good practice always to ask the mother at the appropriate moment 'have you noticed anything about the eyes, is there anything you want to tell me or ask me, are there any eye problems in the family?' It is not unreasonable to propose that most if not all of the foregoing errors could have been avoided by that simple precaution.

THE SETTING FOR THE EXAMINATION

The babies are examined twice, initially soon after birth and again within 24 hours of return home. The first examination is brief; its primary concern is major congenital abnormality or other urgent matters. The discharge examination is more leisured and searching, and indeed it is in the neurological items that the contrast between the two is most obvious. The current vogue for 24-hour discharge is likely to grow; this would probably mean a single routine examination close to discharge.

The examinations are usually done in the nursery with the mother in attendance, but should she be confined to bed the examination is brought to her bedside [24], a natural courtesy that we now understand as beneficial to bonding. It is increasingly the mode for fathers to attend as well. The average nursery is a suitable location; it is quiet and the lighting is usually diffused without glare. A nursery nurse or midwife attends to the baby and also fills in the standard form that is an indispensable part of the examination; this is all good training for her.

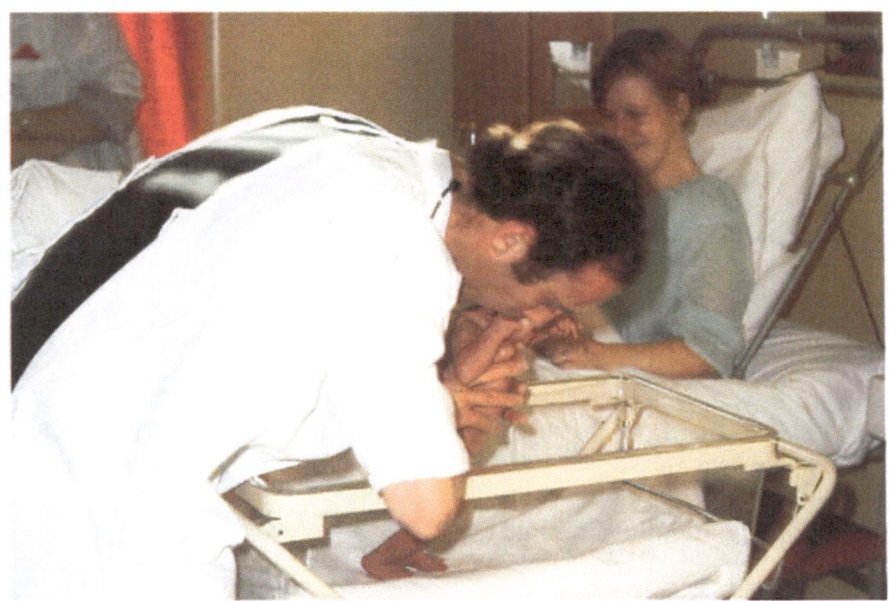

25 A pleasurable encounter

THE BABY'S STATE OF AROUSAL

At birth the baby is usually somnolent, apathetic and hypotonic, which militates against the initial examination. Day by day there is progressive lightening in the level of wakefulness with an actual peak on the sixth day. This concerns only the expert, all we need know is to schedule the definitive neurological examination for the 24 hours prior to discharge and if possible to avoid doing it in the first 48 hours.

More important than daily levels of arousal are the so-called *circadian rhythms* that take place within the course of a day. These have an approximately 4-hourly cycle (they determine the feeding schedule) and there is general recognition of five levels of arousal:

State 5: crying, eyes opened or closed
State 4: eyes open, large movements, not crying
State 3: eyes open, slight peripheral movements
State 2: sleep, light
State 1: sleep, deep

Thus the automaton baby locked in his circadian rhythms is the determinant of the optimal time of examination. In effect, optimal time is between one-half and one hour before a feed is due; the goal, of course, is to achieve dominant state 4 in the course of the examination but, with several babies to be seen in one session, the good primary care doctor soon comes to learn the new skills of shepherding the less biddable babies along the quieter open-eyed path. This is a pleasant achievement [25] that incidentally gives great enjoyment to the mothers and the nursing staff.

AUTOMATIC RESPONSES IN THE PRIMITIVE REFLEXES

An understanding of the baby's physiology is the key to obtaining *seriatim* automatic quieting, eye-opening and widening, then finally side-to-side movements.

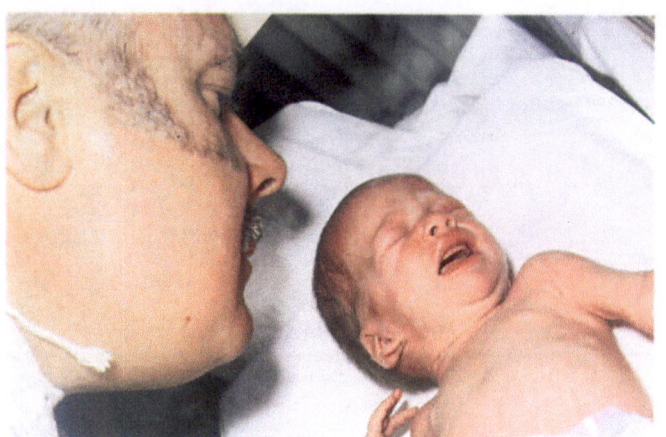

26 Baby in state 5

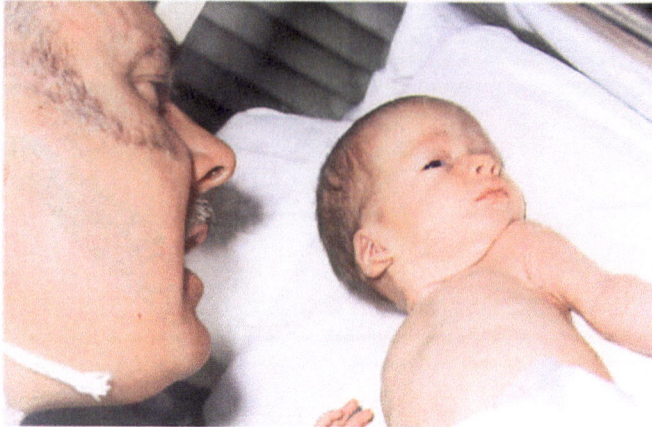

27 Observer vocalizes, baby reverts to state 3

The 'auditory attention' response

This induces quieting and eye-opening [26–28] by a soft 'a-a-a-ah' close to the ear at a rather low pitch. If the baby is fussing with the eyes barely open, the 'attention' response causes wider opening [29, 30] and the eyes often turn to the source of sound.

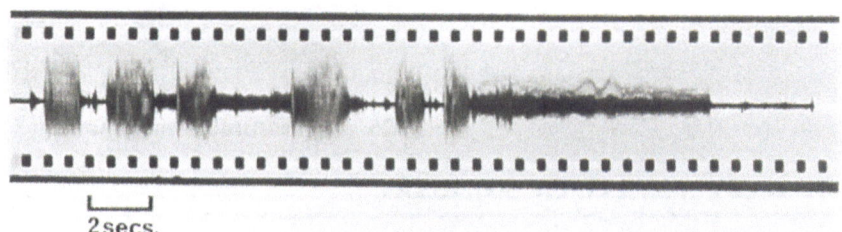

2 secs.

28 Oscilloscope tracing: baby's loud yells are stilled by examiner's soft prolonged vocalization

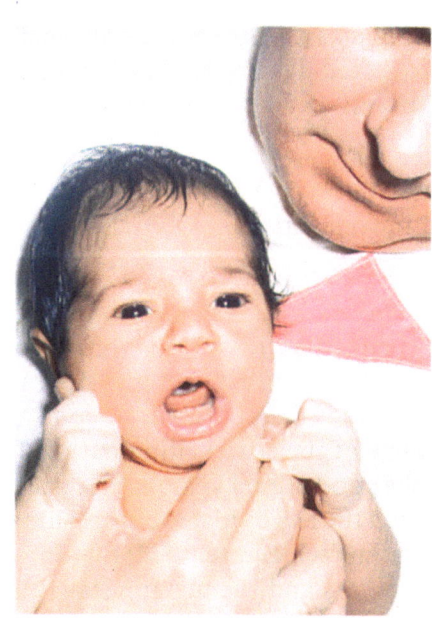

29

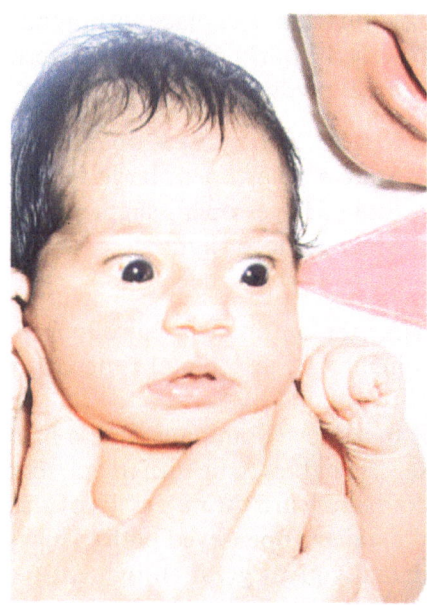

30 A small subconjunctival haemorrhage is revealed (the mother had noticed it) as the eyes turn to the sound and the lids open; note transient 'setting-sun' sign

The automatic sucking response

This reliably produces eye-opening [31, 32] and indeed the quieting–eye-opening sequence is so basic that one constantly sees the babies themselves demonstrate it [33, 34].

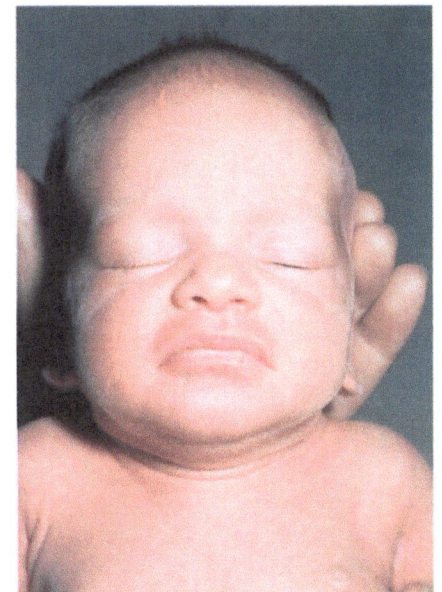

31 Eyes lightly closed . . .

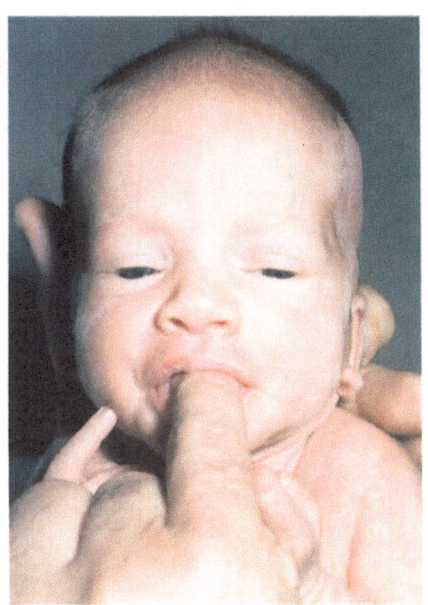

32 Gentle sucking response is adequate

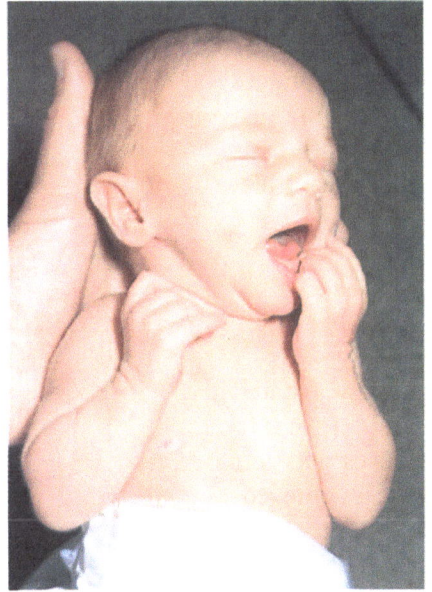

33 A small child . . .

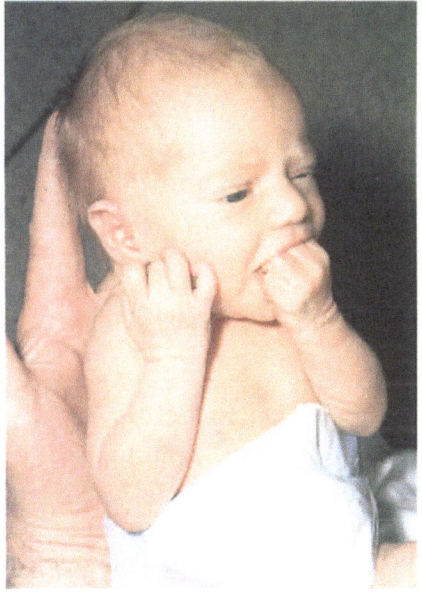

34 . . . shall show you

The 'doll's eye reflex' (upright)

Transition from supine to upright produces opening/widening [35, 36] by a vestibulo-palpebral response with the eyes fixed ahead [and see 55, 56].

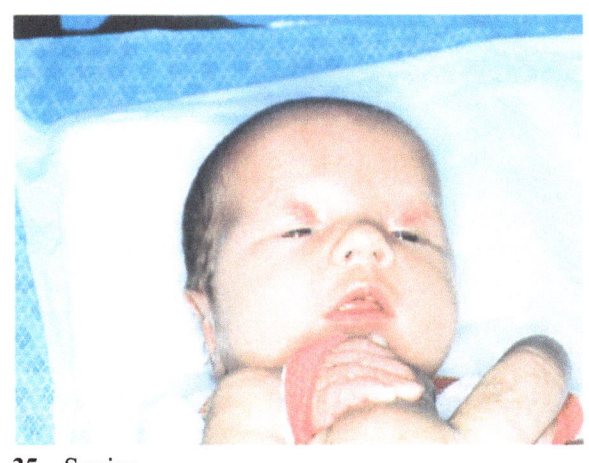

35 Supine

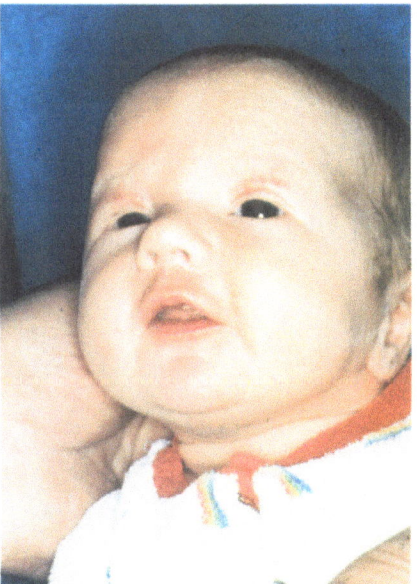

36 Upright

DOLL'S EYE REFLEX (forwards)

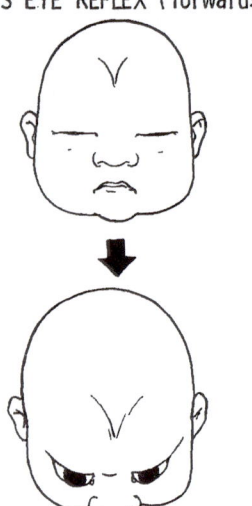

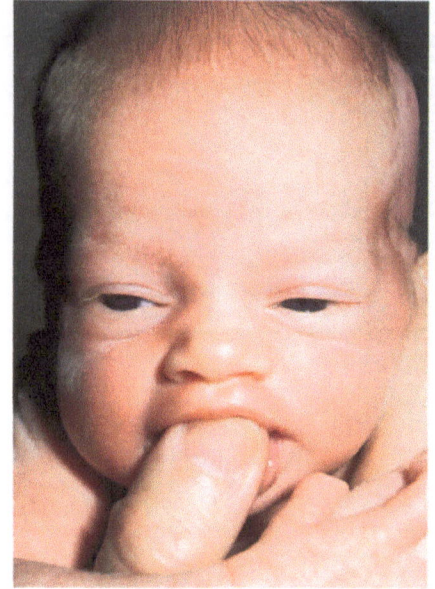

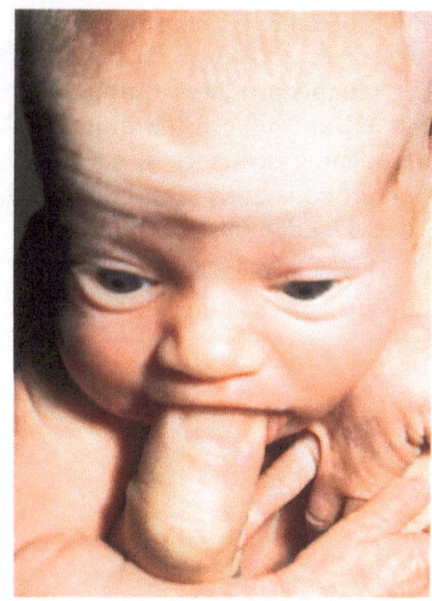

37

38 Upright

39 Tilted forward, note wrinkling due to frontalis action

The 'doll's eye reflex' (forward)

Forward tilting from the upright position produces opening/widening [37–39], gaze ahead is maintained by elevating the eyes, frontalis action elevates the lids and furrows the brow. This is the 'doll's eye reflex' proper, described by Bartels in 1910.

The 'doll's eye reflex' (lateral)

Suspended upright [40] the baby is slowly rotated around the axis centred on his own length [41], first to one side [42] then the other [43]. The eyes get 'left behind' so that the net effect of lateral gaze is achieved. This is too slow to be useful; the eye-turning towards the examiner is a disadvantage.

DOLL'S EYE REFLEX (lateral)

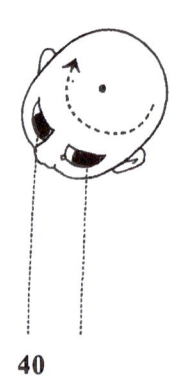
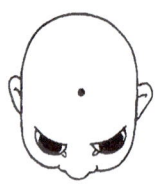
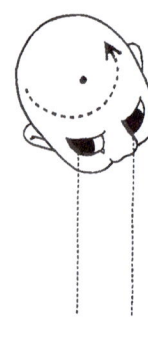

40

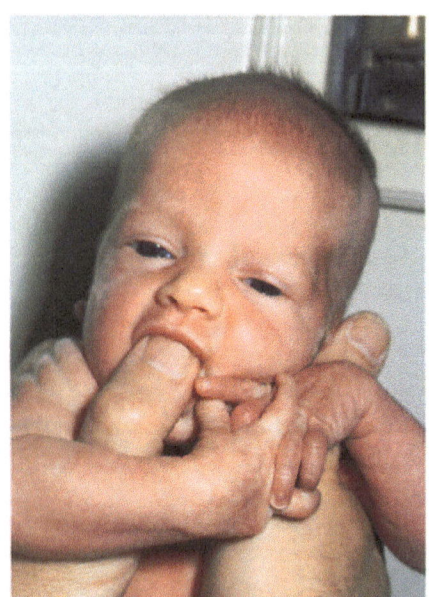

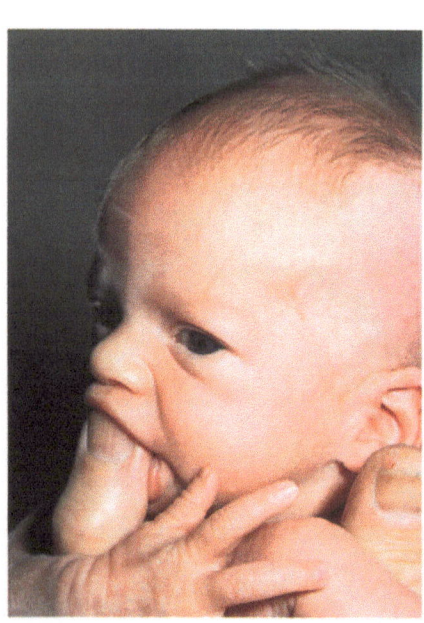

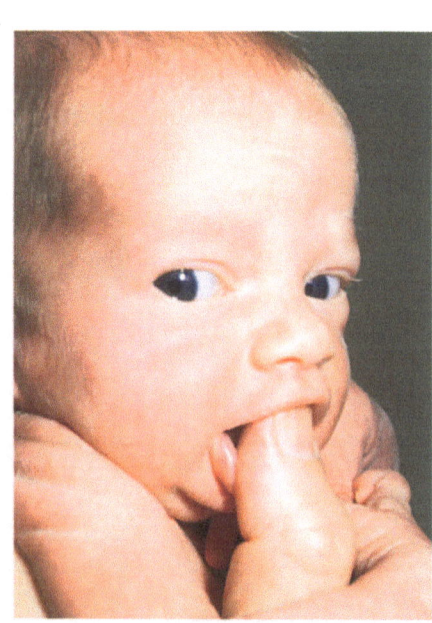

41 Midline position

42 Gentle rotation to baby's right

43 Gentle rotation to baby's left

The labyrinthine response

This is the most important and it is also the easiest. Suspended upright [44, 45] at arm's length the baby is swung deliberately in a 30° arc, first to one side [46], then the other [47]; *once* is enough. The centre of the arc is now in the examiner's body. The main response is that the eyes now turn to the leading side to expose the maximum area of sclera and also reveal 6th nerve palsy where present.

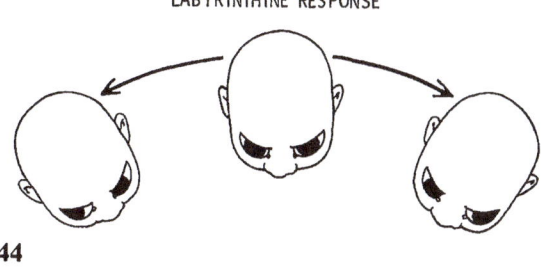

LABYRINTHINE RESPONSE

44

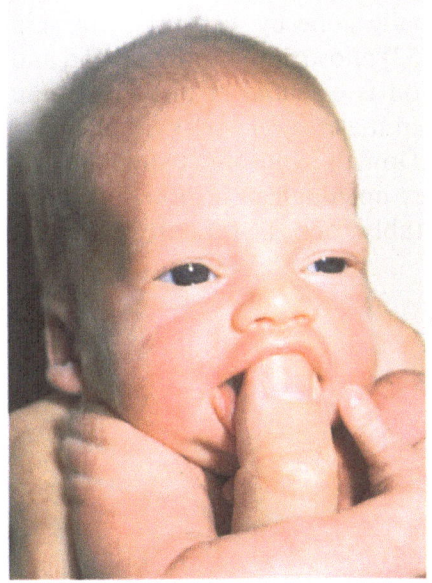

45   Centred

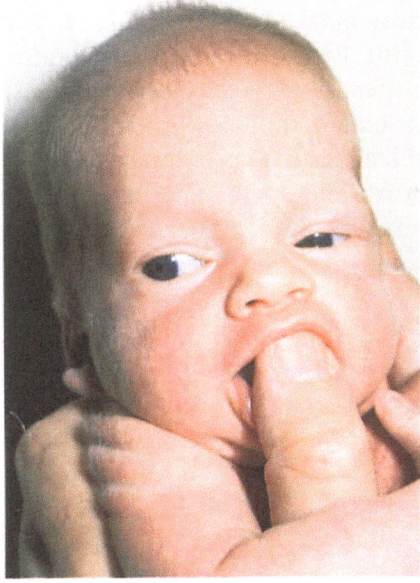

46   Swung to baby's right

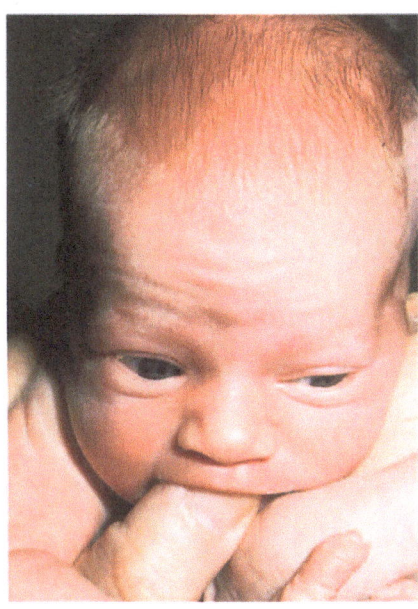

47   Swung to baby's left

Reflex turning to light

This is present in most term babies at the end of the first week. If the baby is simply supported in supine beside a diffuse source of light, he turns first his eyes [48] then his head [49] towards one side, then the reverse [50].

Conclusion

The 'doll's eye reflex' (forward) and the labyrinthine response together are usually sufficient. In practice, a natural flowing sequence soon develops without one's being aware of the components.

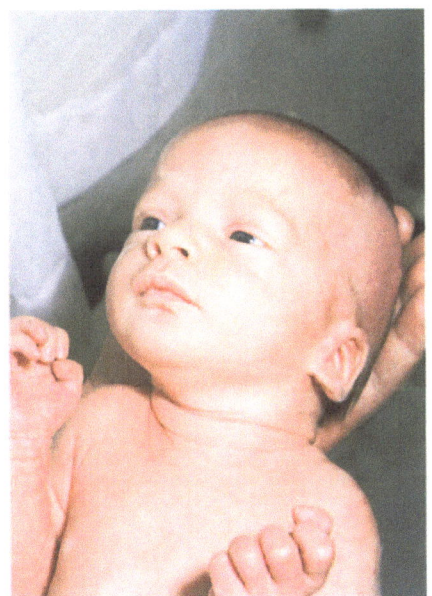

48   Centred

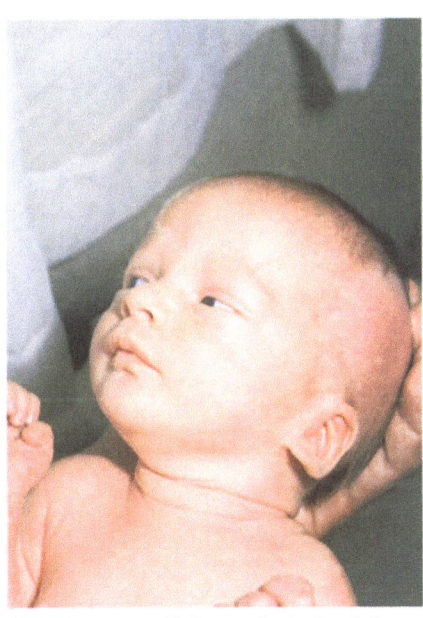

49   Turns to light on baby's right

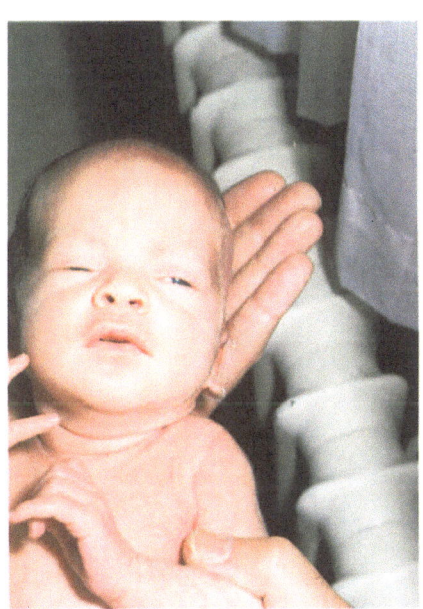

50   Turns to light on baby's left

INSPECTING THE BABY'S EYES

Even after the doctor has employed the baby's automatic responses to achieve wide eye-opening there are a number of conditions that can interfere with the ease of examination and due heed must be taken.

VIEWING PROBLEMS: I. SWOLLEN EYELIDS

Early mechanical oedema is a physiological feature of the first few days, most marked at birth [51]. It has usually gone by 48 hours, but skin naturally lax by race [52] or syndrome [53] allows it to be more florid and to persist longer. When close inspection is essential at birth [54] mild oedema combined with slippery skin can make it very tricky: but here a quick glance was enough to show this Down's syndrome baby had only Brushfield spots. The 'doll's eye' reflex opening can also be interfered with [55, 56] if it has to be done unsuitably soon, as for early discharge home.

51 Within a few minutes of birth only some extreme emergency would make the doctor want to press on and try to force the lids open

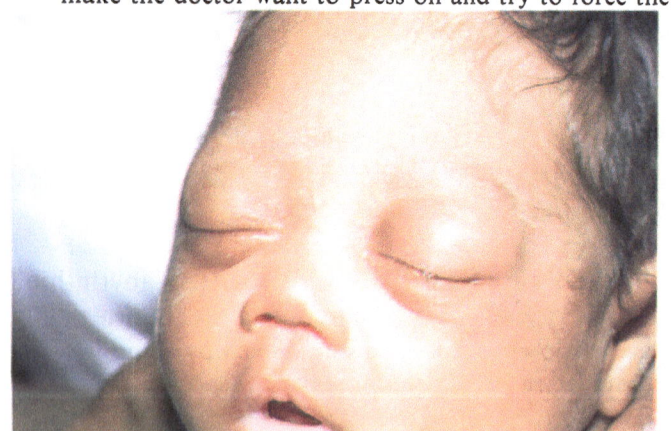

52

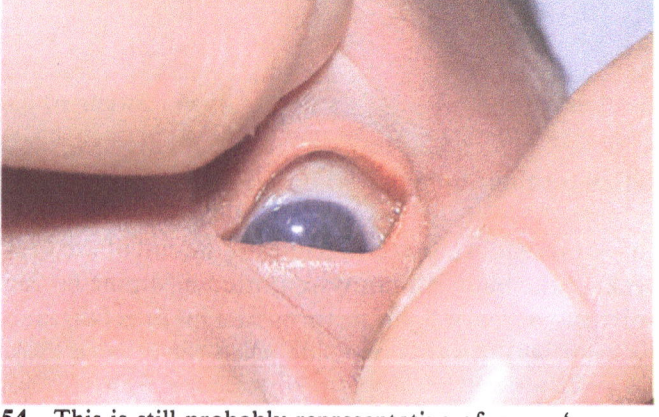

54 This is still probably representative of many 'eye examinations' today

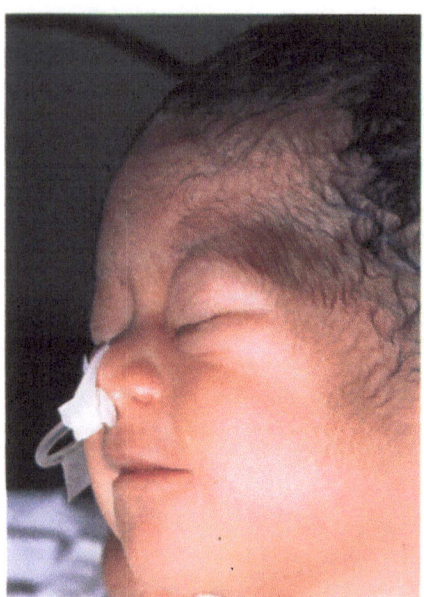

53 Down's half-caste West Indian

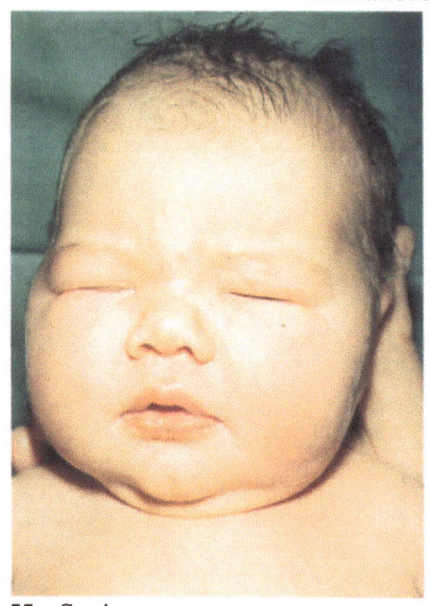

55 Supine

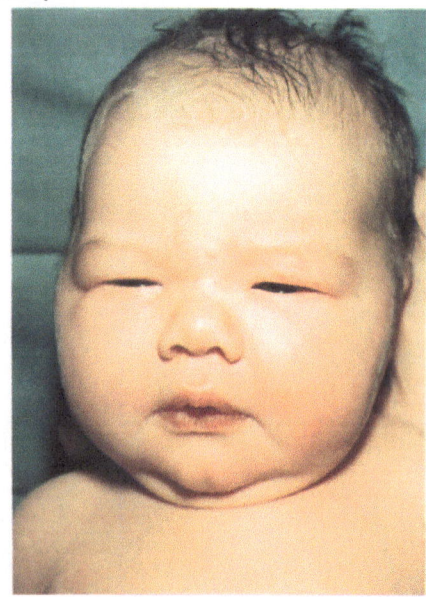

56 Upright

The mechanical oedema of caput succedaneum [57] may be off the face at birth but it can soon gravitate to the eyes and the postural effect [58] can be quite marked. In an apparently similar case [59] the left eye seems *closed*, but in fact it is the right eye that sags open [60] because of facial palsy – caput and facial palsy tend to be linked by the common factor of forceps delivery trauma. When mechanical oedema follows difficult or instrumental [61] delivery the skin often bears the marks, all the more so if there was antecedent caput extending on to the upper face. The post-term baby is in striking contrast [62] with the foregoing; he is conspicuously wide-eyed, having as it were lived out his early postnatal weeks *in utero*.

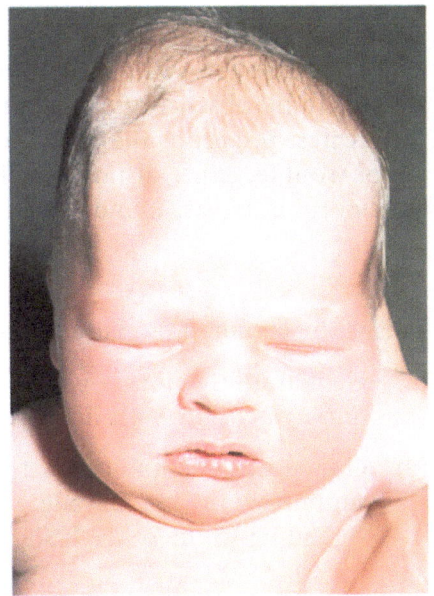

57

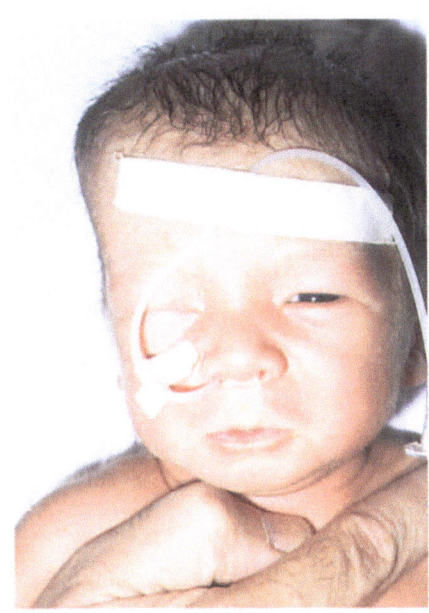

58 Has been lying to the right on a plane surface

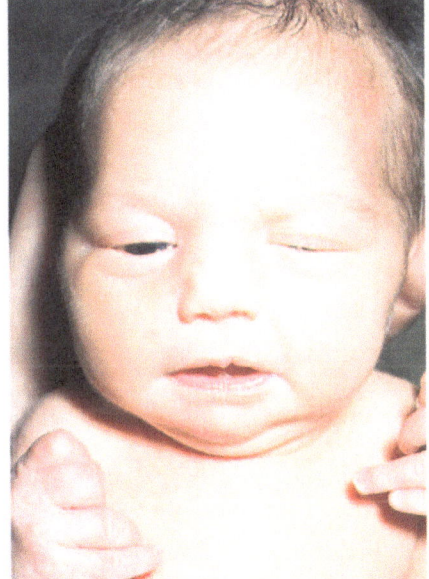

59 Facial palsy at rest . . .

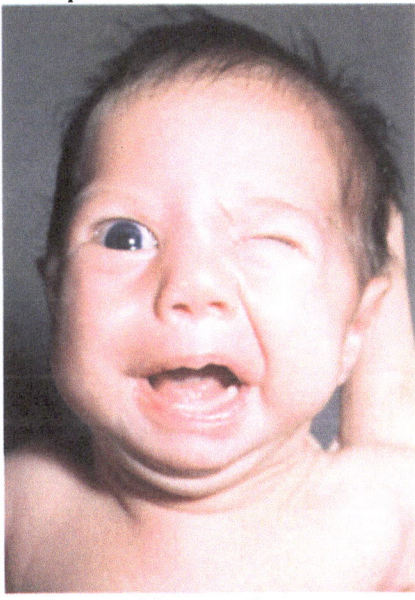

60 . . . And in state 5

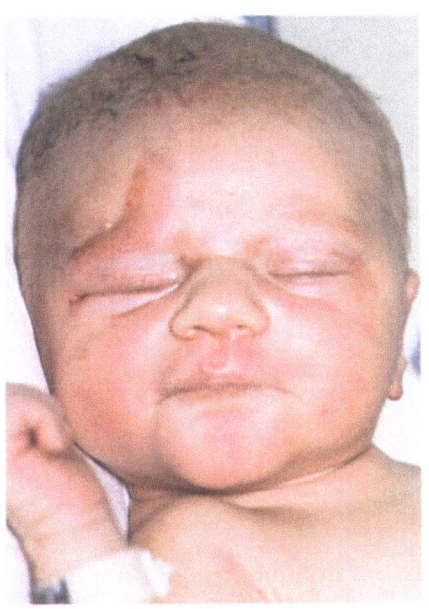

61

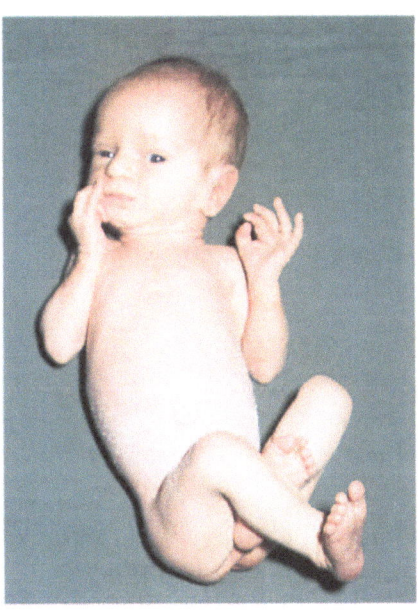

62 Typical long thin baby with peeling skin

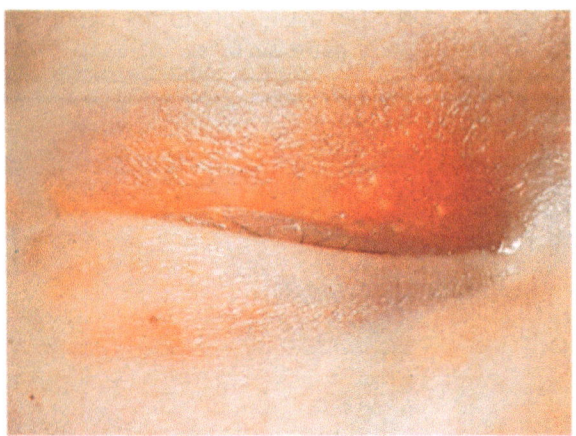

63 Baby looks distinctly unhappy

Pathological swelling

These babies are more or less ill, depending on the cause of the oedema, and of course the swelling will persist if the cause cannot be quickly treated. In the absence of a local cause, swelling of the eyelids commands the greatest respect as the possible non-specific early sign of all sorts of major trouble, either distant or diffuse. In its way it ranks with apathy, circumoral cyanosis, jaundice and mottled skin [63] as a danger signal.

Infection

This is the commonest cause by far.

(1) Neonatal infection is usually with common organisms, especially *Staphylococcus* [64]; lids already swollen are ideal soil for them.

(2) Gonococcal ophthalmia sets up after 3–4 days; there is profuse suppuration, first in one eye where it becomes mature before spreading to the other [65].

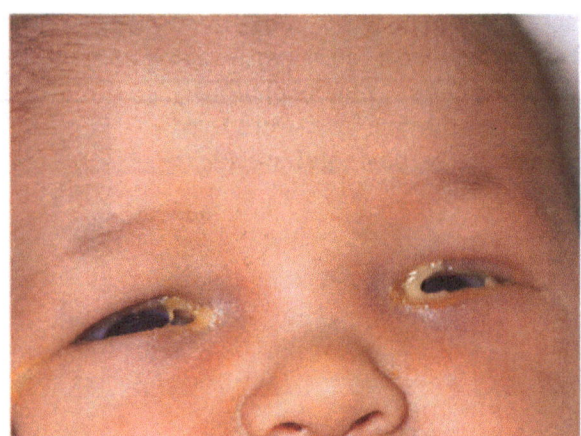

64 Nursery infection is best prevented by the obsessional washing of hands with soap and water between the examinations

65 Gonococcal ophthalmia is more profuse than this in the early stages

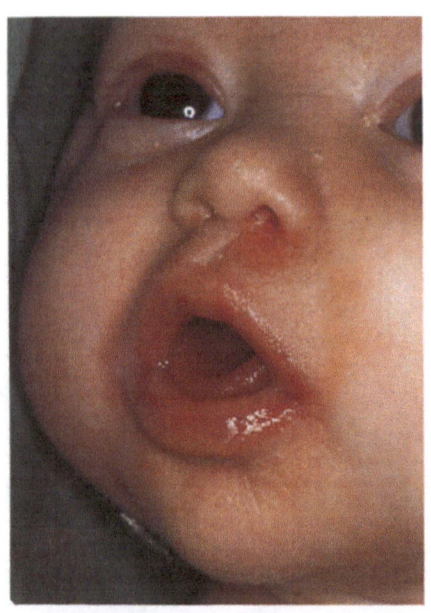

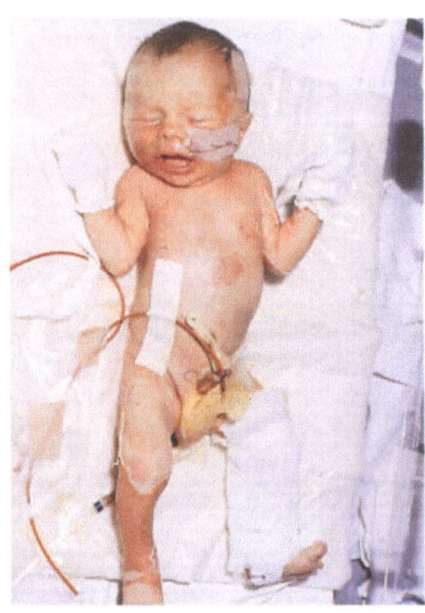

66 Rhinorrhoea (snuffles), extensive involvement responded completely to treatment

67 Infection is cryptic, not in the peeling skin areas

(3) Syphilis deserves inclusion here on grounds of epidemiology, although the usual swelling is in the nasal mucosa due to the characteristic severe rhinitis [66]. Iritis, pallor of the optic disks and 'pepper and salt' chorioretinopathy are common; ophthalmological advice is mandatory.

(4) Distant infection causes swelling of the lids [67]. This is the 'scalded skin syndrome' of Ritter, due to staphylococci, phage type B.

Various skin disorders

These cause lid swelling in an incidental way: congenital ichthyosiform bullous erythroderma [68], epidermolysis bullosa [69], Bloch–Sulzberger incontinentia pigmenti [70], and the baggy redundant skin of cutis laxa (Ehlers–Danlos) [71], for instance. In one case of 'collodion skin' due to lamellar ichthyosis [72], the severe change has caused ectropion in addition. The prognosis is excellent: half recover completely, the other half have lamellar ichthyosis, usually mild in degree.

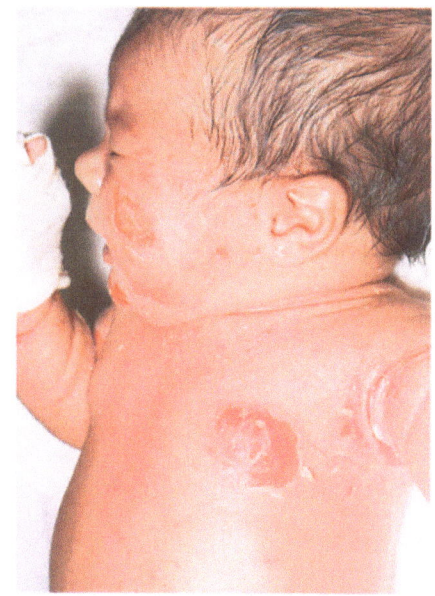

68 There are always some thickened skin areas to be found on careful search

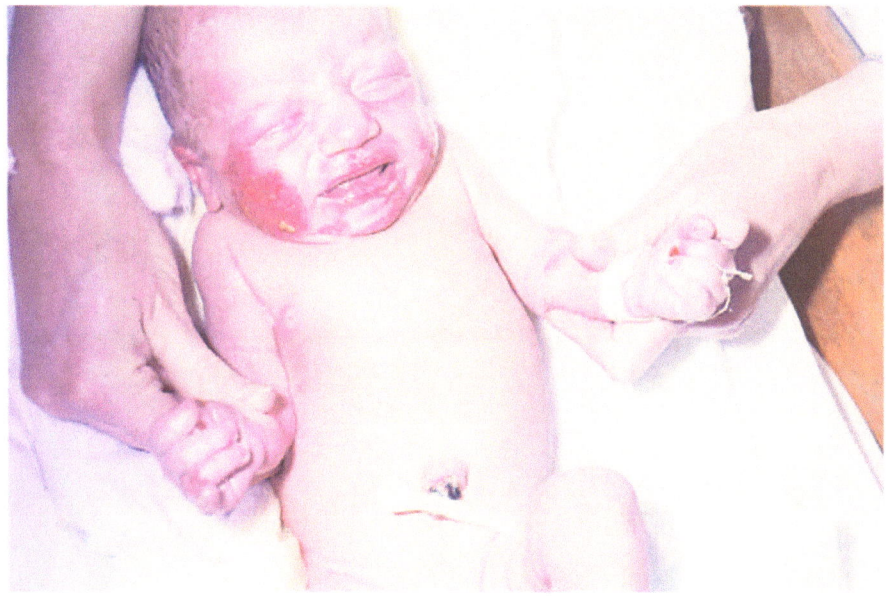

69

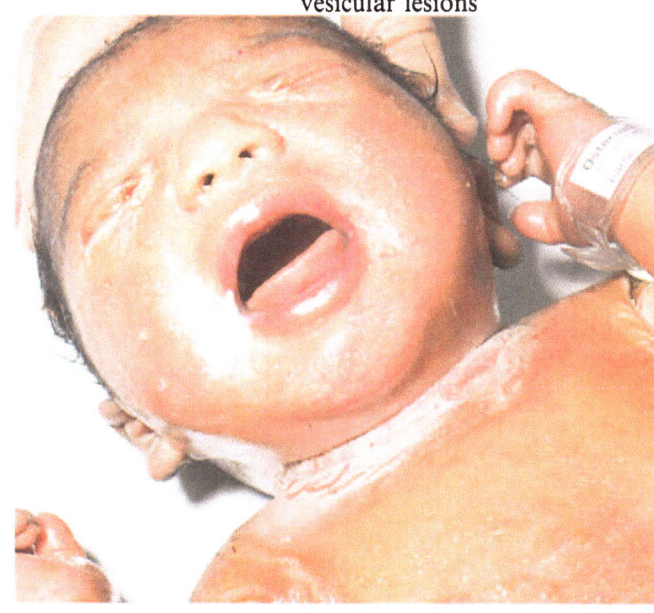

70 There are almost always a few vesicular lesions

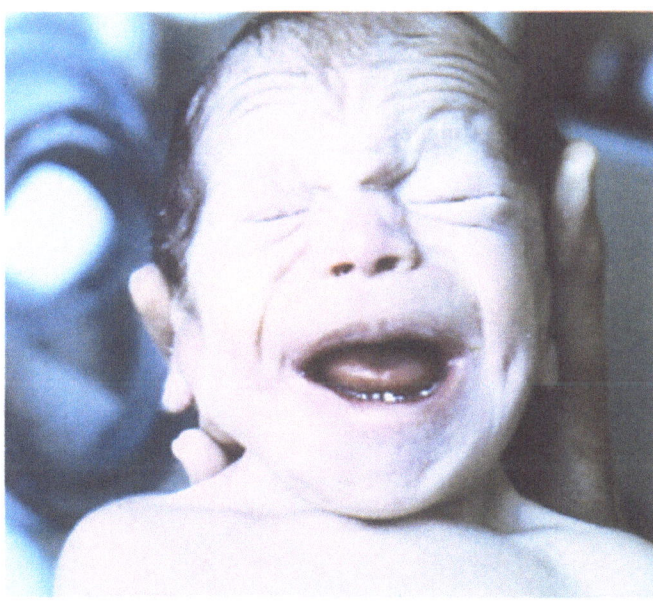

71

72 The lids are everted

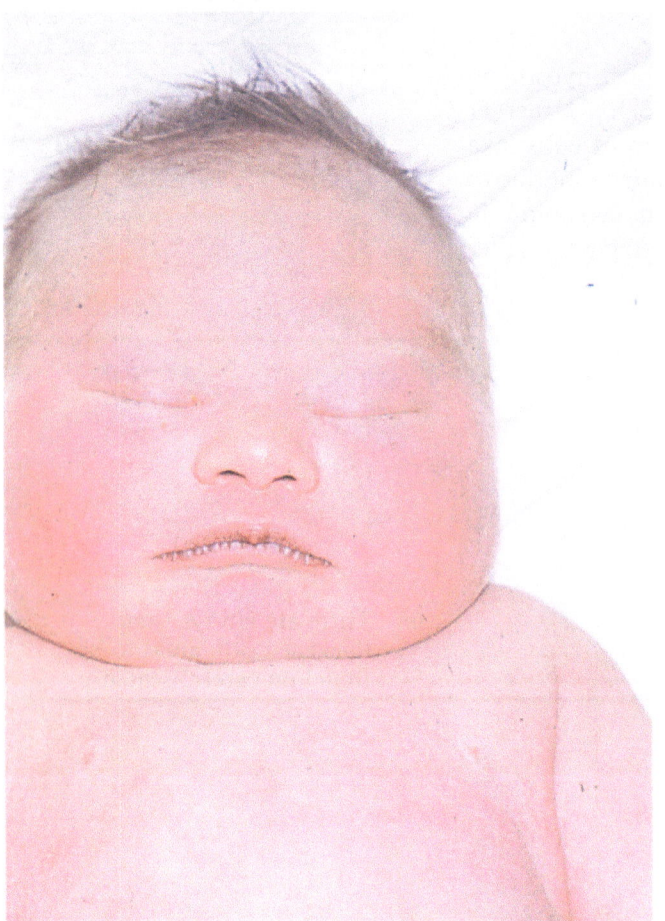

73 Round head and short neck are typical additional clues

Circulatory disorders

Heart failure can cause oedema of the face and lids: in the first case [73] shown here, the baby has Down's syndrome and a peculiar 'ballerina' touch to the upper lids; in the second [74] the oedema impedes lid opening but a few Brushfield spots can be glimpsed in the left eye; this is *not* Down's syndrome, a reminder that these spots occur in 10% of all infants.

Thyroid disorders

Congenital hypothyroidism [75] can cause eyelid 'myxoedema' that may persist for weeks [76]. This is perhaps better known as a historical feature of cretinism in later infancy [77], when it can be of considerable degree but is by no means invariable [78]. Routine histochemical screening for congenital hypothyroidism has shown a substantial number of cases without swollen eyelids [79].

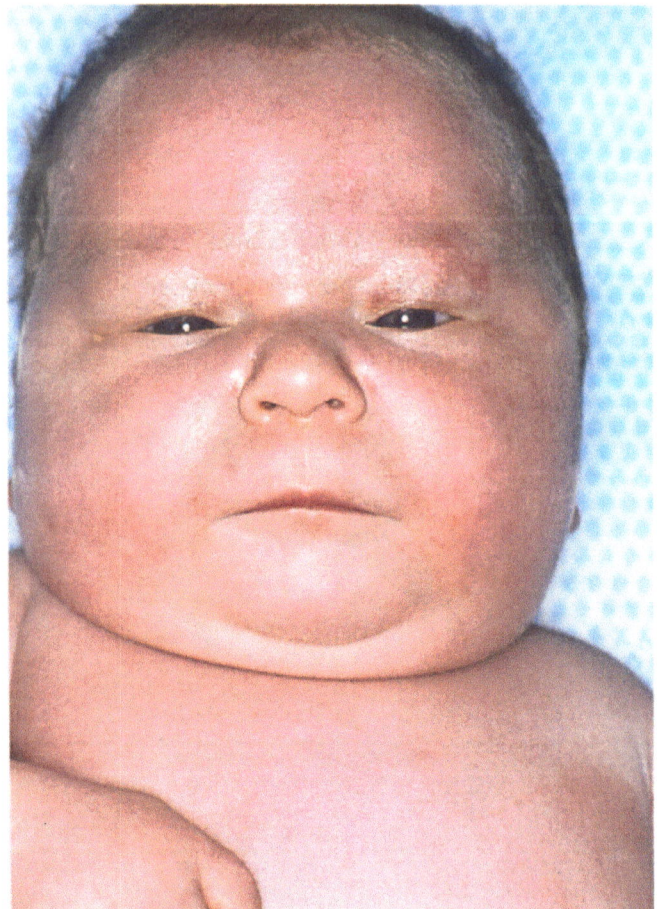

74 A more alert looking baby

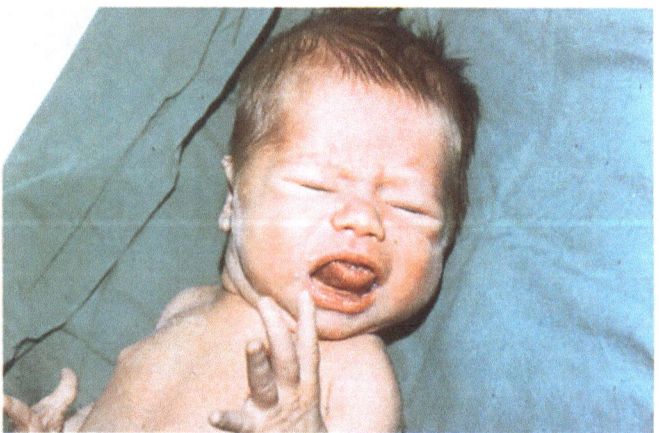

75 Note large tongue . . .

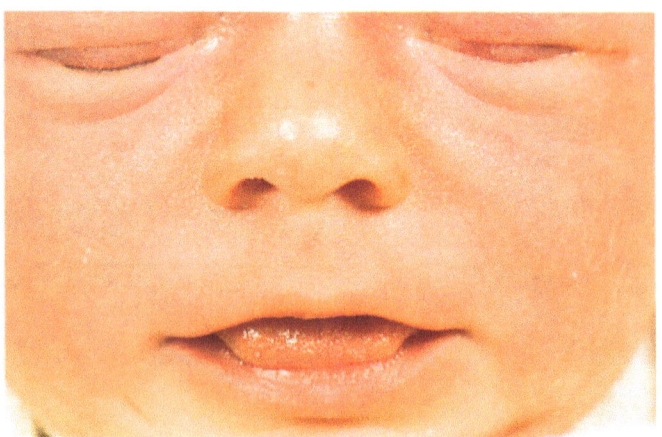

76 Two weeks old, skin still looks rather coarse

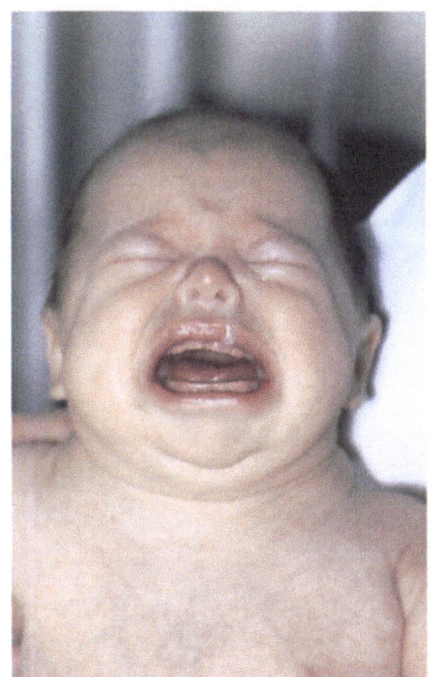

77 Note nasal secretions, supraclavicular pads and mottled skin

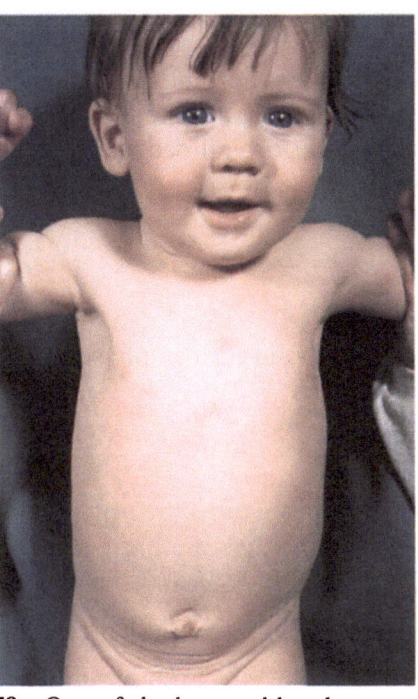

78 One of the better old-style patients, with screening this is now the rule

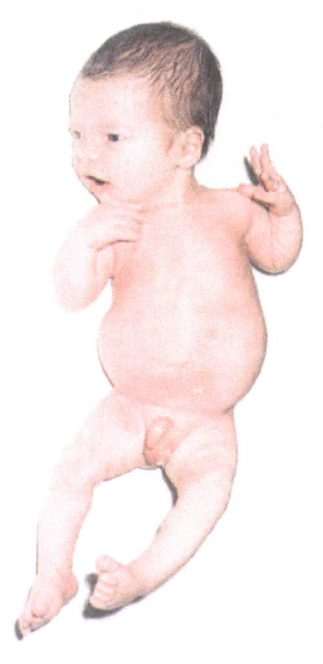

79 Typical contemporary case found on screening

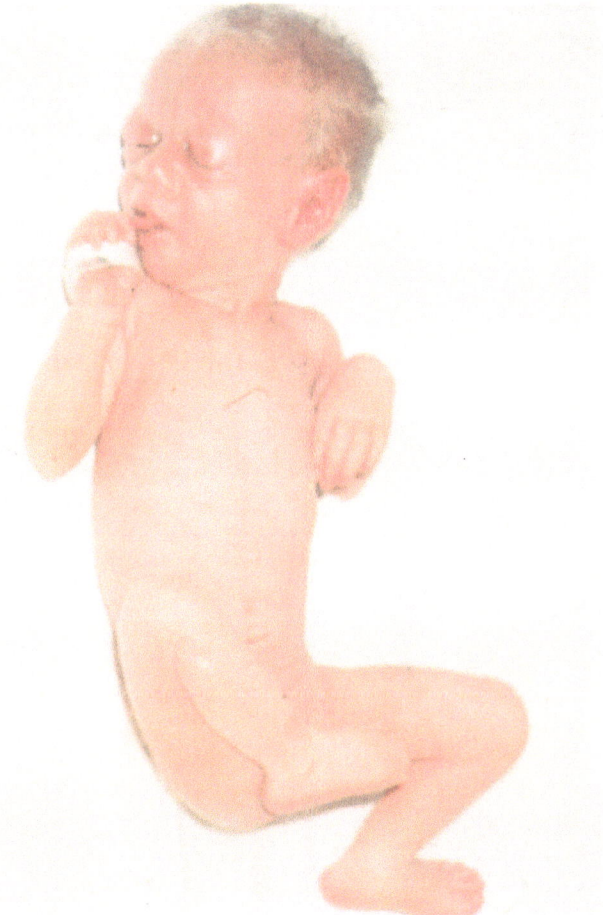

Congenital hyperthyroidism [80] in one case showed very swollen eyelids; it could be that the situation was aggravated by *chemosis* (oedema of the conjunctiva). An extreme example of chemosis [81, and see 373] was seen after assisted ventilation in a baby with Apert's disease.

80 Jittery hyperactive baby, fetal heart rate constantly over 120 per minute

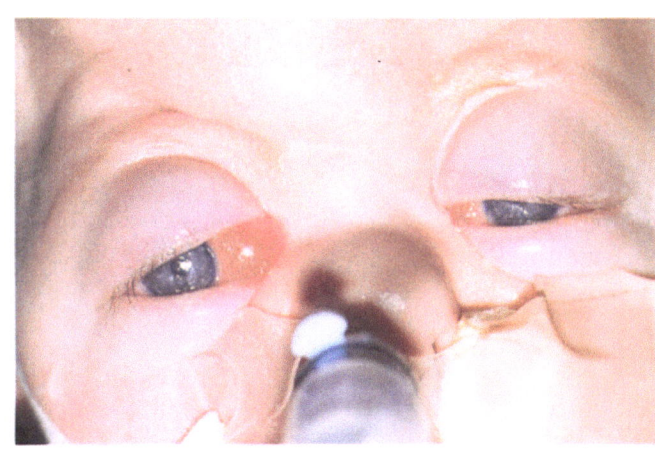

81 Apert's disease, chemosis (conjunctival oedema) on ventilator

Severe generalized oedema

This may occur in hydrops, congenital nephrotic syndrome or with severe liver pathology [82]. The ballooned facial appearance is quite stereotyped.

On the other hand, an occasional case of periorbital oedema remains unexplained even though it persists for weeks [83].

Iatrogenic

In a unique case the swelling [84] was caused by surgical emphysema due to attempted jugular venepuncture.

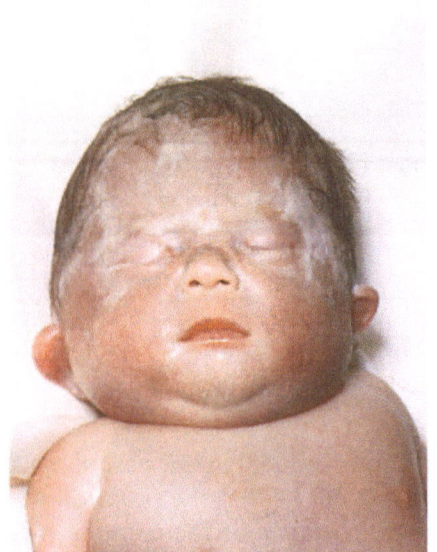

82 Severe liver disease with low serum albumin

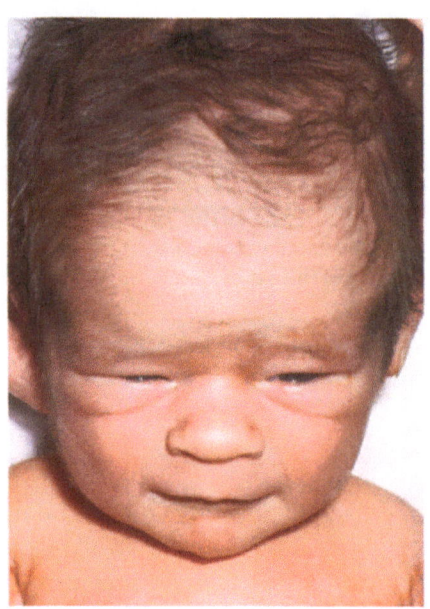

83 Oedema unexplained

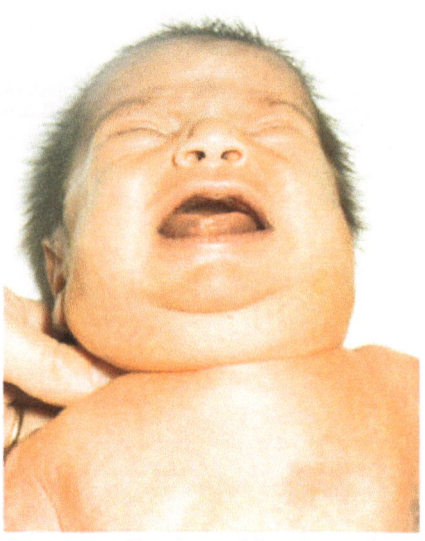

84 Complication of jugular vein puncture

VIEWING PROBLEMS: II. ABNORMAL EYELIDS

Ptosis is the commonest by far [85]; it is usually of mild degree but neuro-muscular conditions like myasthenia gravis or myotonic dystrophy should be kept in mind. In cases of ptosis with lid deformity [86] there may be a small cyst that requires surgery later [87]. In one instructive case 'mild' ptosis was the indicator of unexpected minor neurological dysfunction in the nursery. There is moderately severe developmental delay with autoid behaviour [88] and partial trisomy 15 has been discovered. In its context 'mild' ptosis can no more be disregarded than 'small' cataract.

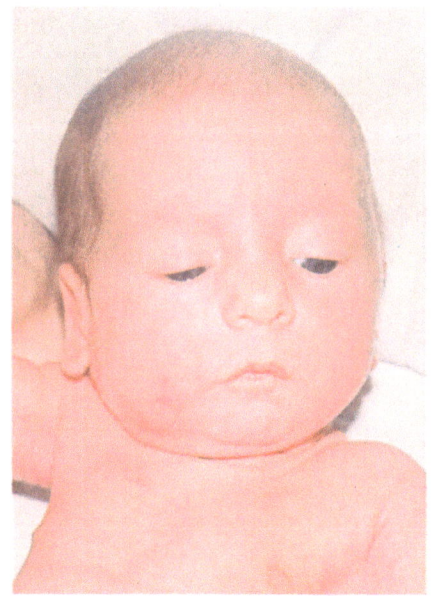

85 Unilateral ptosis . . .

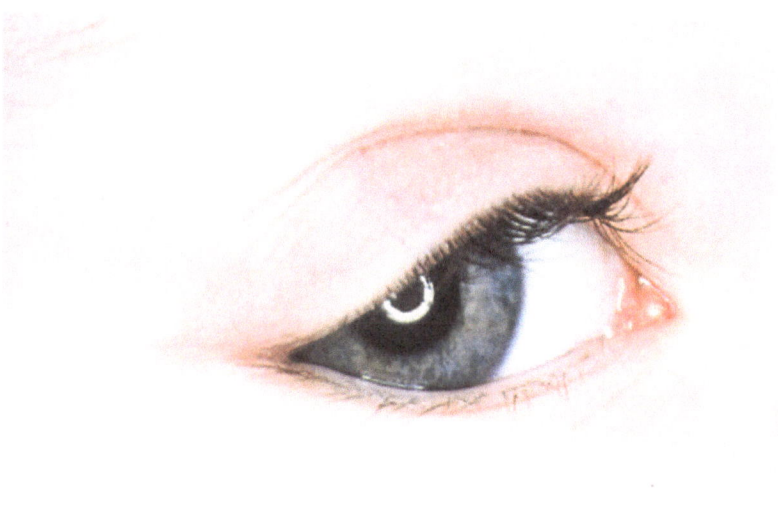

86 . . . Swelling in lid . . .

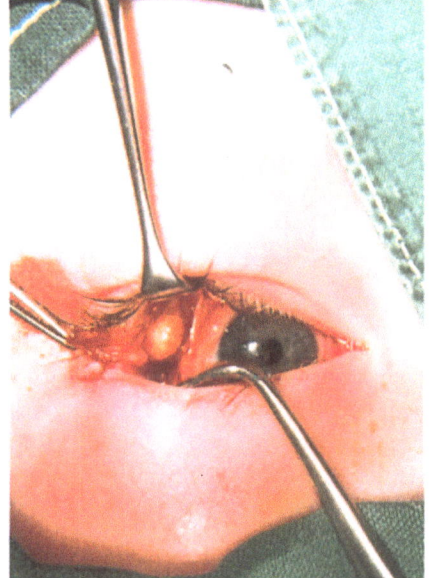

87 . . . Excision of small cyst

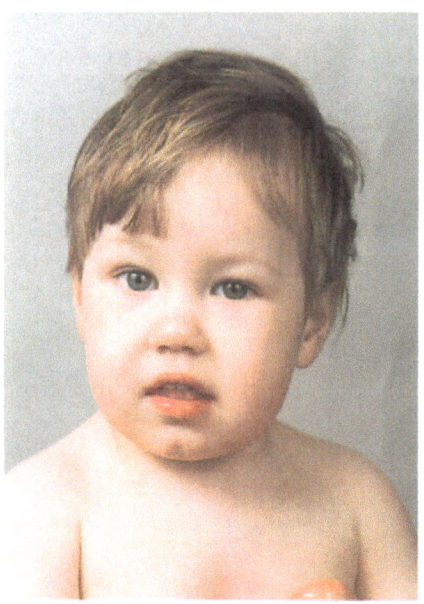

88 A boy who became 'autoid' later on

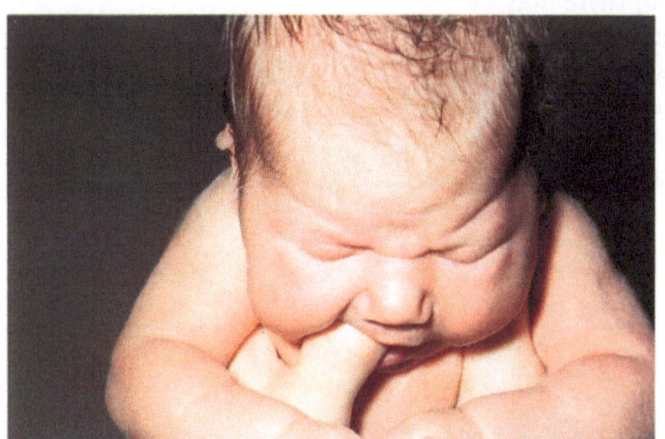

In one instance 'bilateral ptosis' [89] fully resisted reflex opening in the nursery and there was little improvement by 6 [90] months. Long before then we knew that he too had inherited the familial condition [91] of *blepharophimosis* from his mother [92], so he was referred to the family ophthalmic surgeon. The facial appearance is initially unflattering and may suggest impaired intelligence; in fact the IQ range is 75–100, mean value 85 and there may be trisomy-20p. In moderate cases of ptosis [93], the decision is usually for plastic surgery, for cosmetic–morale reasons.

89 Complete failure of doll's eye reflex forward manoeuvre

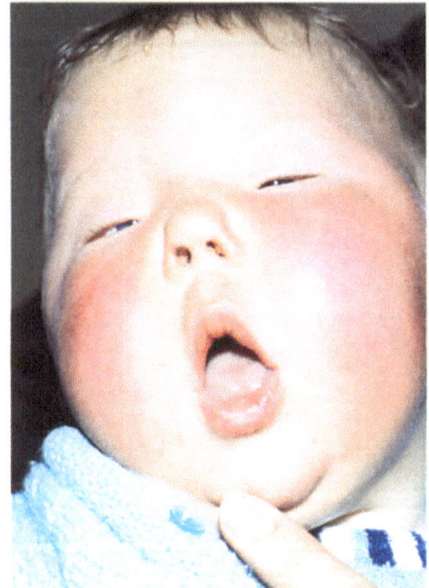

90 Blepharophimosis

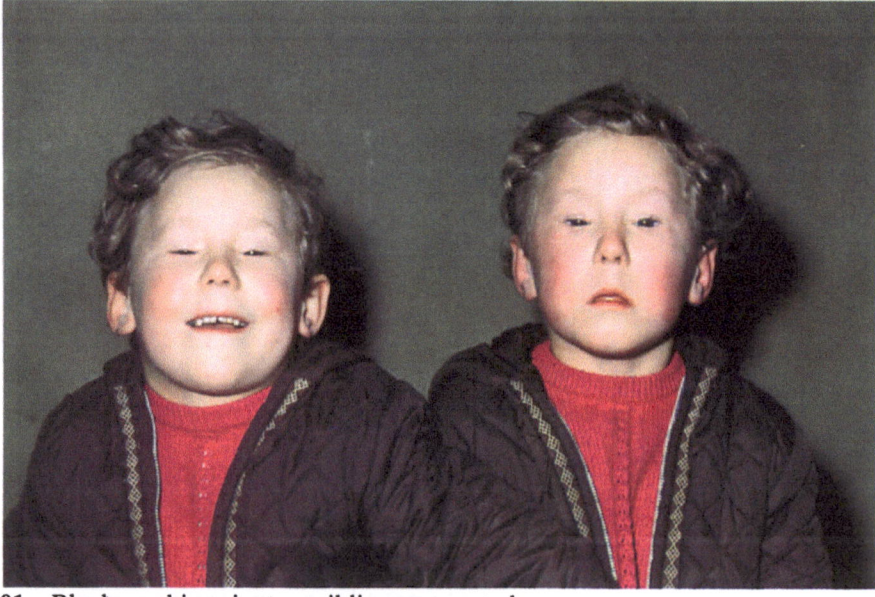

91 Blepharophimosis, two siblings, operated

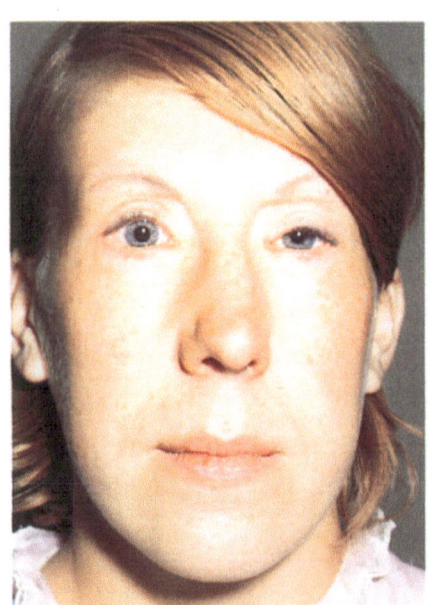

92 Mother, operated

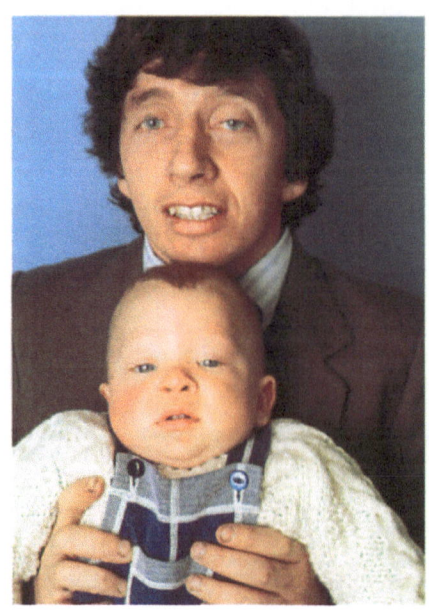

93 Father has been operated

Sometimes congenital ptosis is affected by the jaw movements of sucking [94, 95]; this is the Marcus Gunn jaw-winking phenomenon, an innocent curiosity which clears up spontaneously.

Children may screw their lids up to 'squint' if bright light affects them in albinism [96, 97], cystinosis [98, 99, 21], aniridia [see 219] or dysautonomia [see 290], for instance.

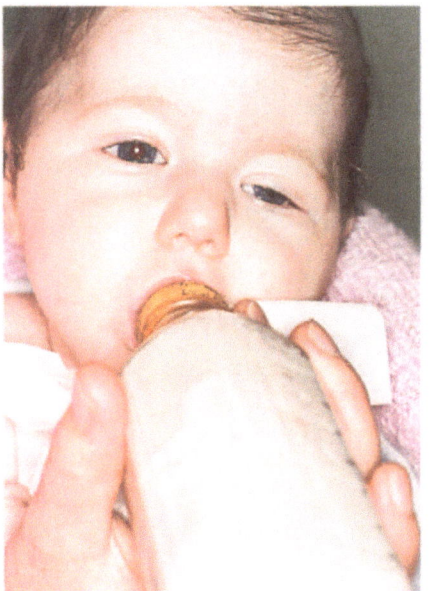

94 Marcus Gunn . . .

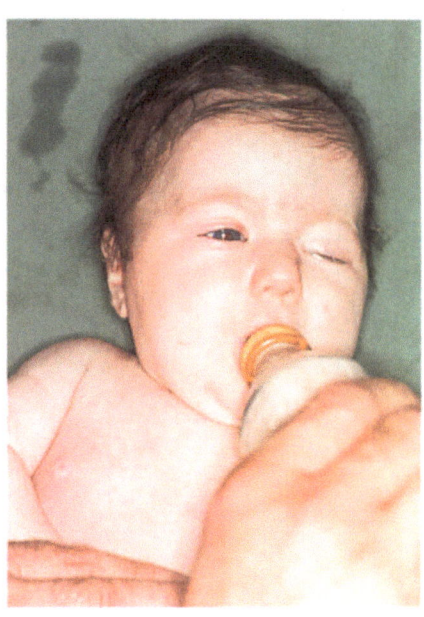

95 Jaw-winking phenomenon

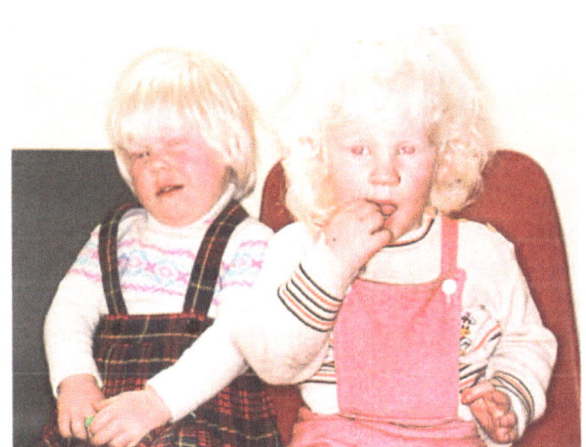

96 The arrival of the second albino was a surprise?

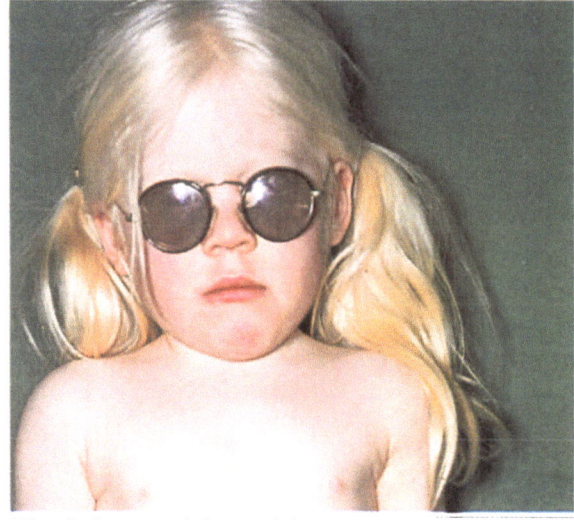

97 Only one girl opted for sun glasses

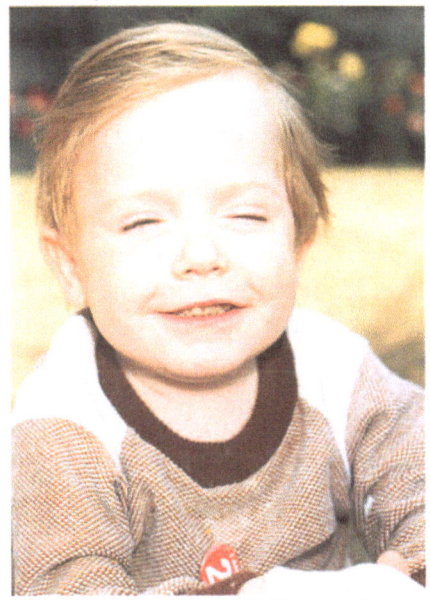

98 Cystine crystals diffract light to cause glare, like dappled sunlight on water

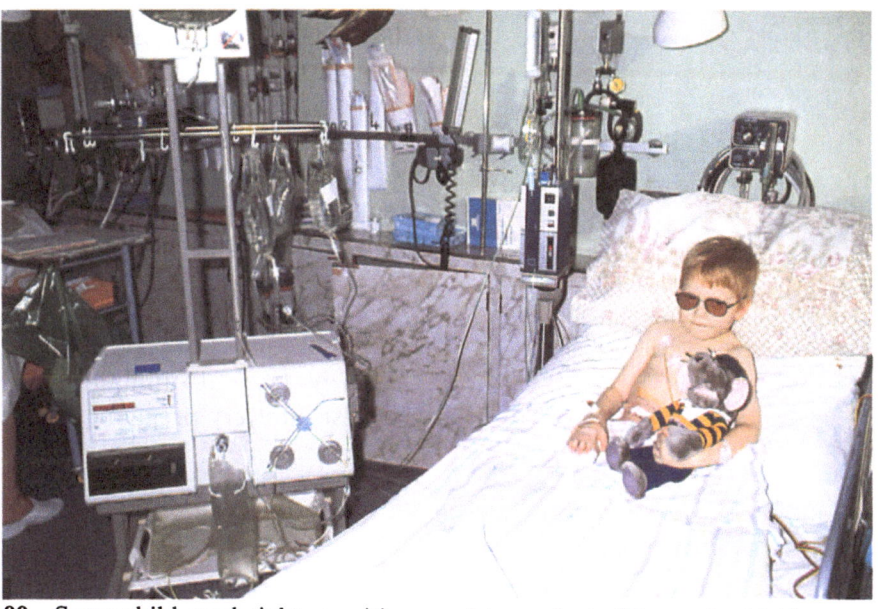

99 Same child aged eight, awaiting renal transplant, this can be highly successful

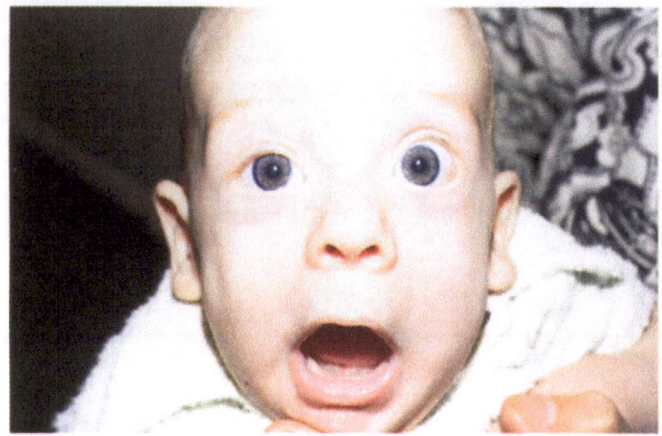

100

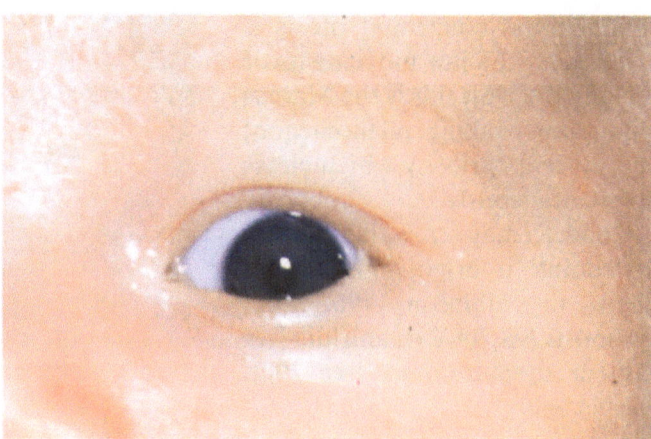

101 Single band across palpebral fissure

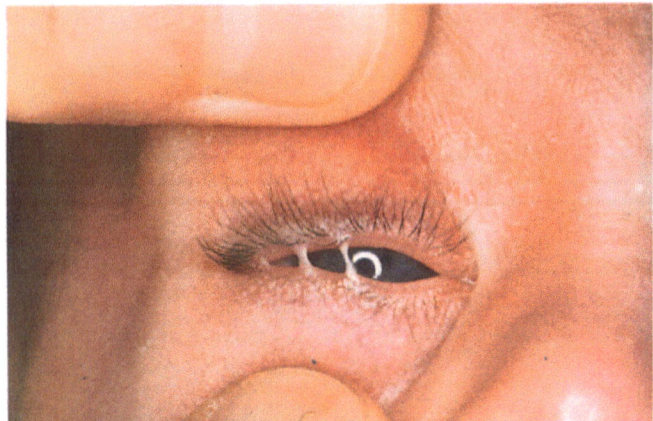

102 Bridges of highly extensile . . .

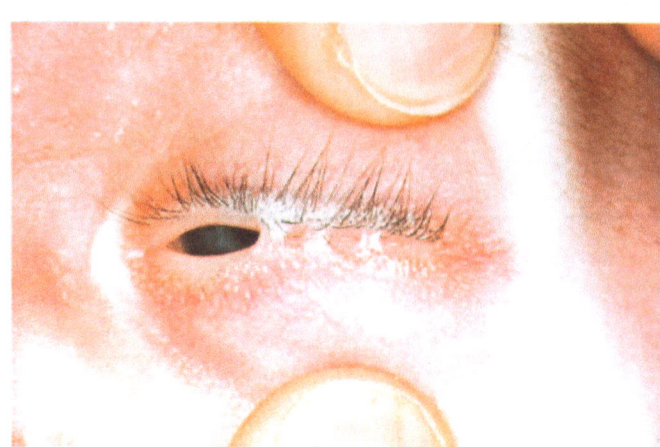

103 Tissue across the palpebral fissures at birth

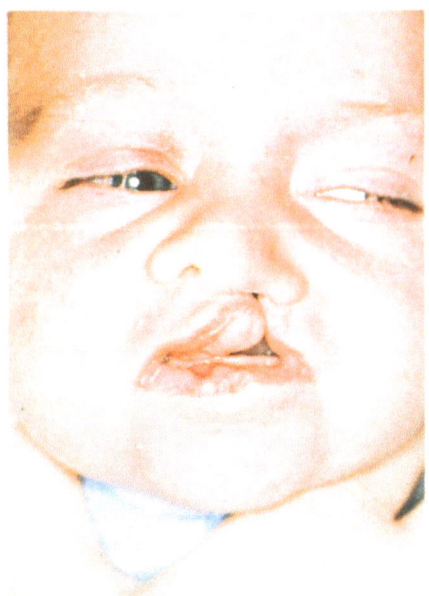

104 Ankyloblepharon may be associated with hair-lip, note some bands still present

Unilateral wide opening may be seen in sustained retraction of the upper lid [100]; here it is exaggerated by mouth-opening, through the so-called 'spreading reaction'. These two acts of extension are mutually interactive, as every dentist knows.

Bridging of the palpebral fissures may be so mild as to escape notice [101] or it may be severe [102, 103], this latter is *ankyloblepharon filiforme adnatum*. The lids themselves have separated but the palpebral fissure is bridged by strands and bands of tissue that is quite elastic, easily stretching to double its resting length.

The severe form is rare but frequently associated with facial clefting [104]; curiously there is no eponym for this combination. Some of the bands dissolve spontaneously and their complete surgical dispersal is a simple matter [105] that is better done in the nursery. The eye itself is spared any lesion. If in addition there is ectodermal dysplasia [106] it is then named the *Hay–Wells 'AEC' syndrome* (Ankyloblepharon, Ectodermal dysplasia, Clefting).

Genetic advice is interesting.

(1) *Ankyloblepharon with cleft*: in 31 cases reported only one had an affected sibling (by history) so the risk is low.

(2) *Hay–Wells*: Dominant inheritance, so an affected parent has 50% risk in every pregnancy. There is partial sweating; IQ is normal.

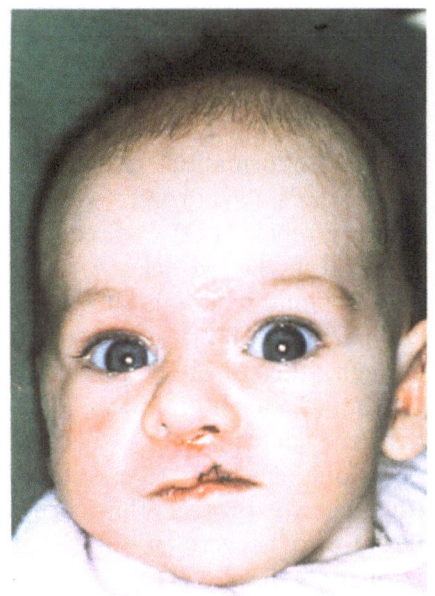

105 Lip repaired, bands snipped

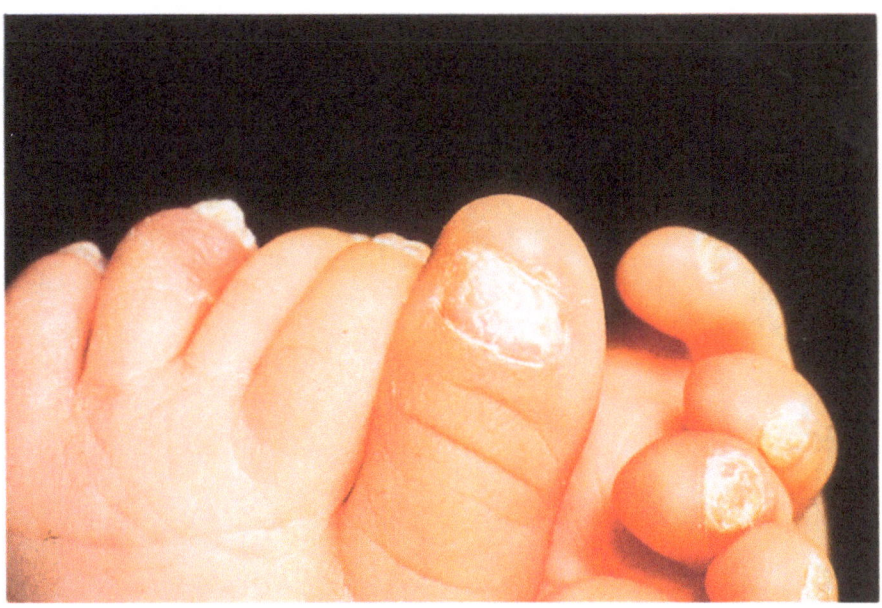

106 On the day, the general skin was clear but there was still ample evidence in the toenail dystrophy

Unyielding lids may conceal anophthalmos, here bilateral [**107**] in a rubella baby, unilateral [**108**] and unexplained in another case. Prostheses are inserted as soon as possible, certainly by age 3 months; young babies accept them readily and facial deformity is minimized [see **9, 10**]. The lids may also resist opening in cases of microphthalmos [**109**]; this baby has trisomy-13, severe ocular pathology is common.

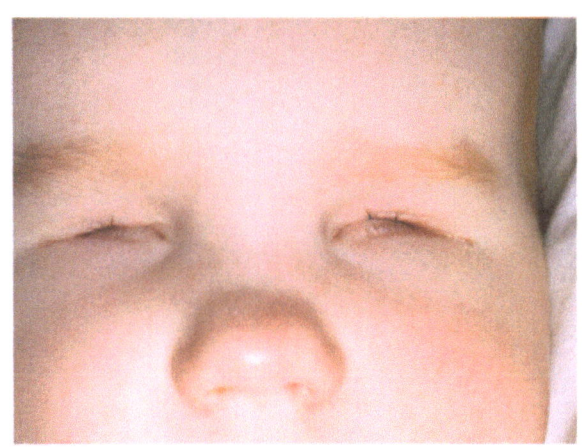

107

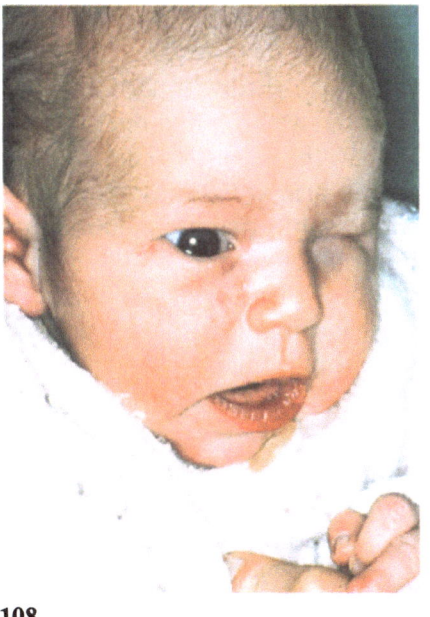

108

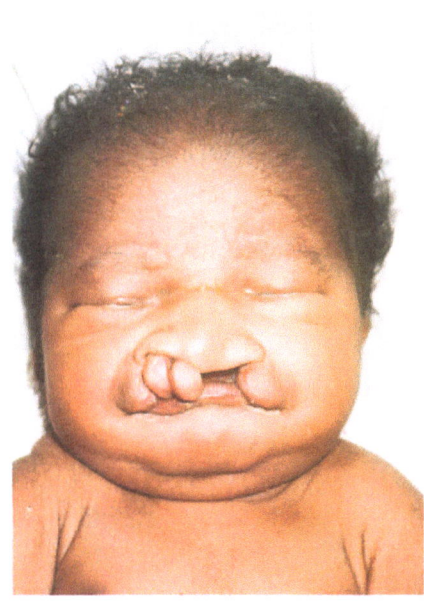

109

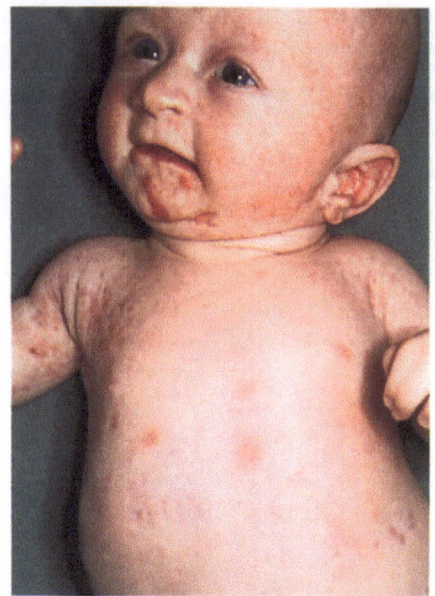

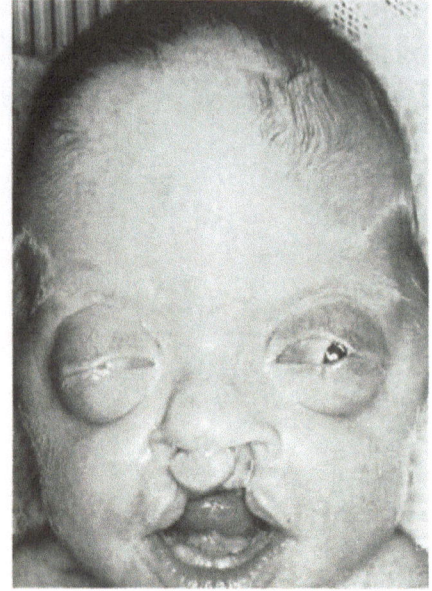

Finally, *any widespread disorder* may by chance involve the lids [110]. This is focal dermal hypoplasia with excrescences and skeletal abnormalities reminiscent of Goltz's syndrome; urgent primary repair [111] was required to protect the cornea. A more typical Goltz's baby is shown for comparison [112]; interestingly enough, this disorder can cause coloboma, itself a focal ectodermal defect. On another occasion the lids had to be stitched together to protect the cornea because of severe proptosis in Crouzon's disease [113].

110 Note excrescence on right cheek, deformity right hand

111

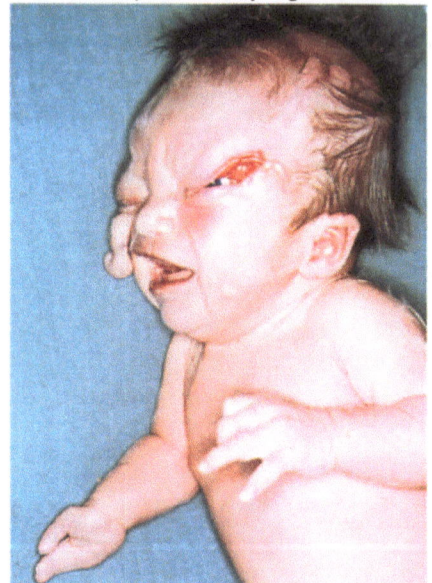

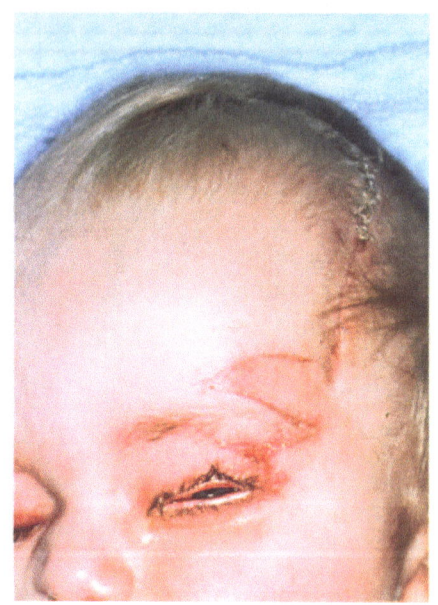

112 Multiple small skin defects, herniation of fatty tissue commonly occurs

113

THE IRREDUCIBLE MINIMUM OBSERVABLE

When I worked with Dr Pamela Zinkin in the newborn nursery at Guy's Hospital we both had research experience in clinical neonatal neurology. We saw the need for a simple reliable neurological examination to be done by the primary care doctor and set about devising one. This excluded subtle subjective items and kept to simple objective ones. The willing junior doctor could do the examination up to a good level of reliability, within the course of 5 minutes, after a few days' part-time teaching.

Accordingly, in the matter of examining the eyes some classical items such as pupil size and reaction to light were self-excluding from universal observation and we were left with those now described.

EYES

The items are:

(1) Straight/constant deviation of gaze

(2) Squint

(3) Subconjunctival haemorrhage no/yes

(4) 6th palsy no/R/L

(5) Other

The first four items must always be recorded, these are functional; the fifth leaves an open field, usually for structural anomalies; everything else is a bonus.

As a matter of interest, if unequal pupils *were* to feature under (5), it would probably be in Horner's or Möbius syndrome, so the ocular observation would be secondary to a remote nerve lesion and not properly in the province of the primary examination of the eyes.

Straight/constant deviation of gaze

Eyes straight

The axes are very nearly parallel, except in extreme lateral gaze or when the baby is tired. It can be difficult to be sure sometimes, especially if there is a prominent epicanthic fold or a broad root of the nose (telecanthus). The corneal reflections of light solve this problem; they are quite symmetrical [114] when the eyes are straight. This is well shown [115] in a baby who happens to have neurological dysfunction characterized by right hemisyndrome. (The *corneal reflections of light* are not to be confused with the *corneal reflex*, an unpleasant measure guaranteed to disturb the baby and precipitate him rapidly into State. 5; it is properly reserved for adults but still features in some paediatric texts.)

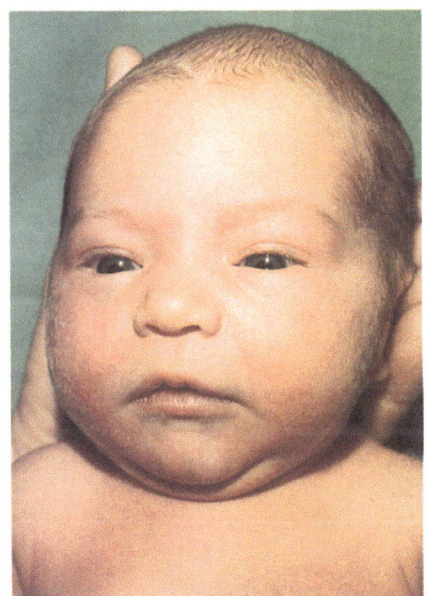

114

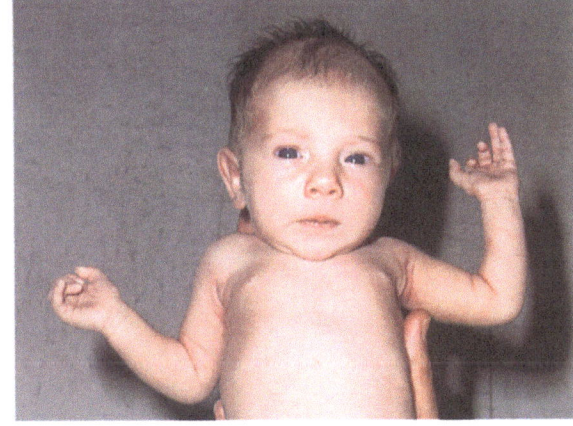

115 Right-sided hemisyndrome, note right upper limb falls away

Constant deviation

The baby is centred throughout on the main source of light whether supine or upright. If the eyes at rest look away from the forward direction this is *deviation*, it is constant if maintained for more than 30 seconds in State 4 or 5 (cf. the rule of thumb measure of time for defining strong Asymmetrical Tonic Neck Posture); the onus is on the tutor to teach reliability in this one slightly subjective item where anyway the borderline case is a rarity. An additional quality of *staring* is soon noted, it comes from the combination of intensity and lid-retraction [116, 117] and their gaze is *unseeing*. These babies had signs of neurological dysfunction.

Deviation forward

This is a fixed gaze ahead that does not wander to either side [118]; this baby is also staring. Her skin rash is that of incontinentia pigmenti, a neuroectodermal dysplasia that may include cerebral malformation [119].

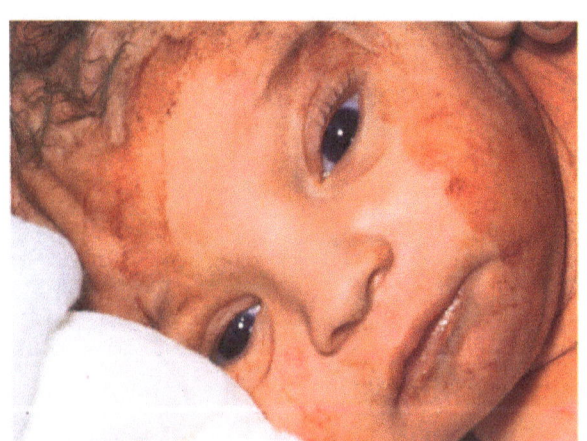

116   Age 1 hour

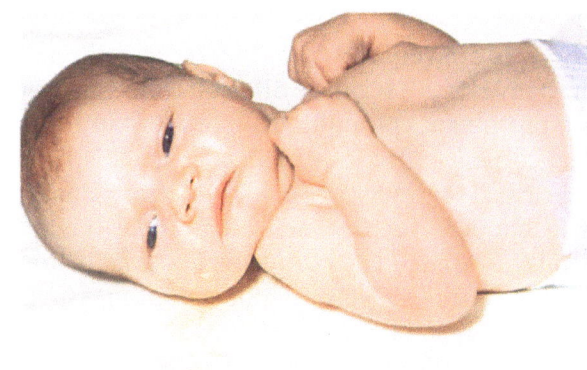

117   Age 2 days

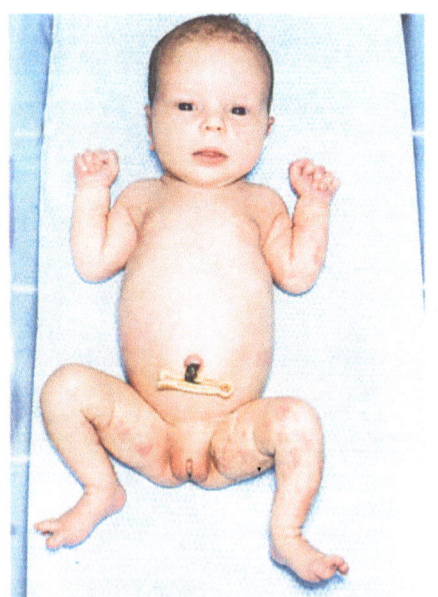

118   Skin eruption of incontinentia pigmenti, note frog position and fisting

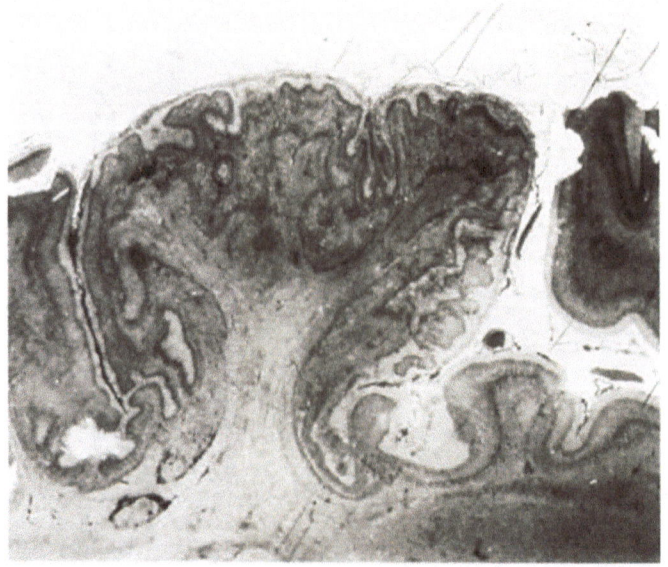

119   Polymicrogyria

Deviation downward

This eventually exposes sclera above the iris, the notorious 'setting sun' sign. Every student knows its historical association with kernicterus [120] and hydrocephalus [121], both now treatable by preventive measures. Formerly, the kernicterus survivor was liable to choreoathetoid cerebral palsy, and he then might show failure of *upward* gaze. When hydrocephalus is relieved [122] the setting sun sign goes away, but this may take quite some time. In this instance sunrise occurred by the age of 3 months [123, 124], and longer persistence than this is regarded as serious, whatever the underlying causes.

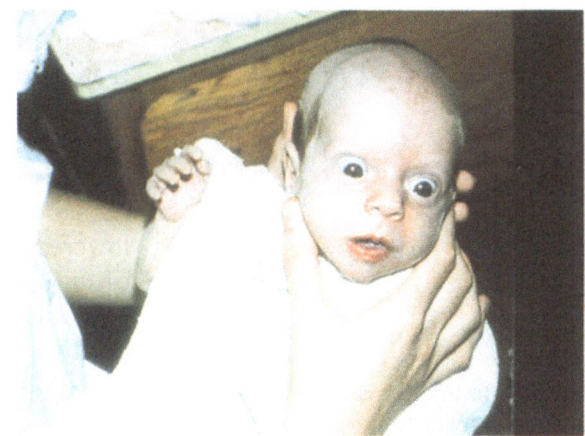

120 Hyperbilirubinaemia resolved, postkernicterus

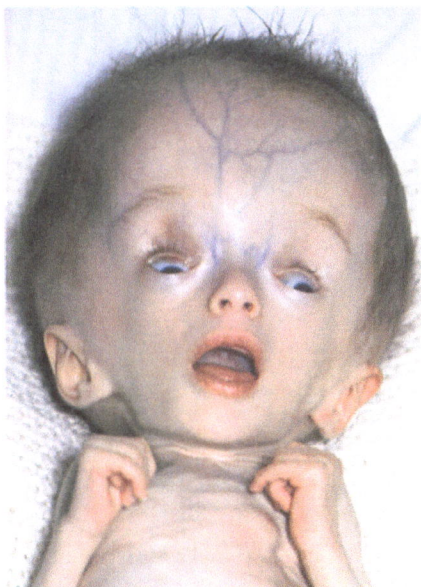

121 Unoperated – multiple malformations

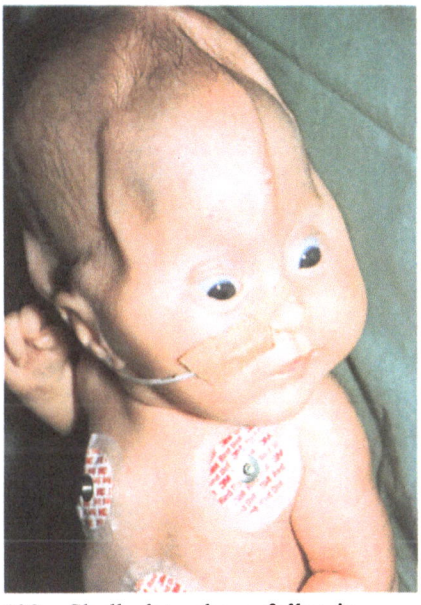

122 Skull plates have fallen in, note 'setting-sun' sign

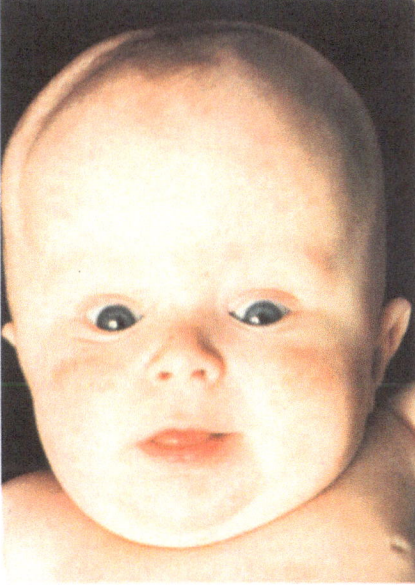

123 Gaze is almost but not quite horizontal in this picture . . .

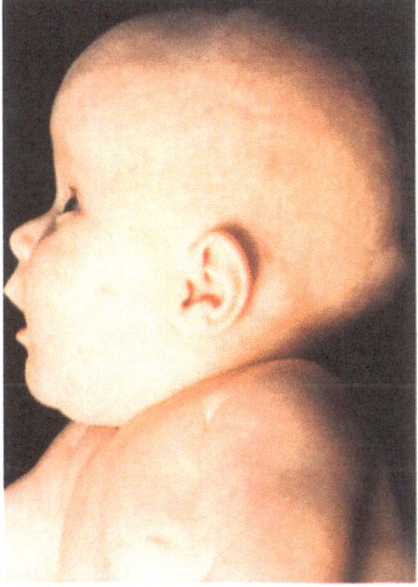

124 But the lateral view shows that some upward deviation is possible

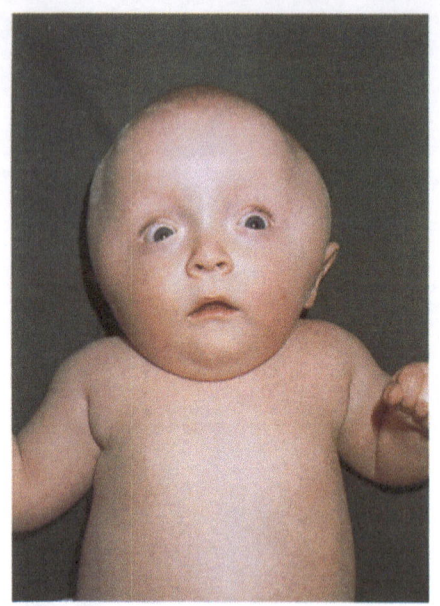

125 Note low-set ears turned downwards

In a young infant with multiple cranial synostosis the sign was observed [125] while the ventricular volume was still normal [126]. The response to surgery was prompt and at 5½ years head size is 75th centile and school progress is normal. The degree to which the 'setting sun' sign is seen in minor neurological dysfunction, especially hyperexcitability states [127], has been understated, and it may persist for many weeks. It has been seen with hyperthyroidism [see 244].

Some normal babies [128] also show it, especially on rapid transition from supine to upright – the *'doll's eye reflex' (upright)* stimulus. It is stronger in the preterm and there may be conjugate deviation inward. In term babies it is gone by 1 month, in the preterm it persists longer [129]. There is an *'eye-popping reflex'* of normal young infants, the palpebral tissues widen suddenly and forcefully if the ambient lighting level is lowered abruptly. The positive response is highlighted by the appearance of an upper scleral rim (25% in the neonatal period) and the younger babies have downward gaze as well; it was invariably present in the 8% positive in the newborn nursery.

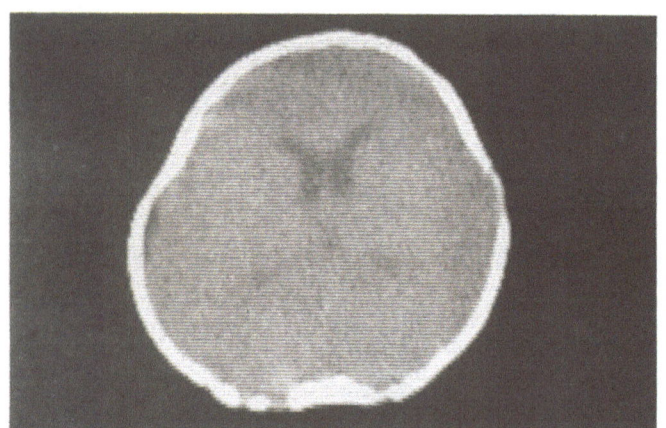

126

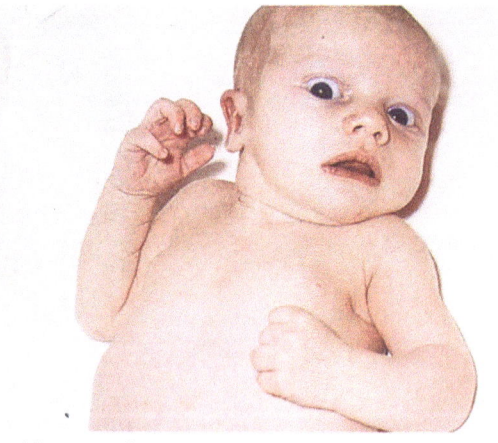

127 Note anxious expression

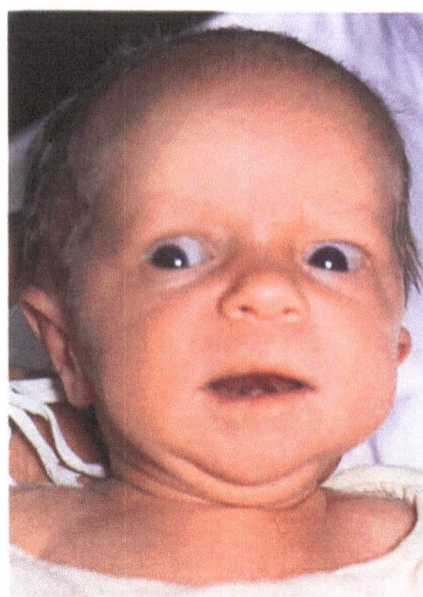

128 Note right eye turned down slightly

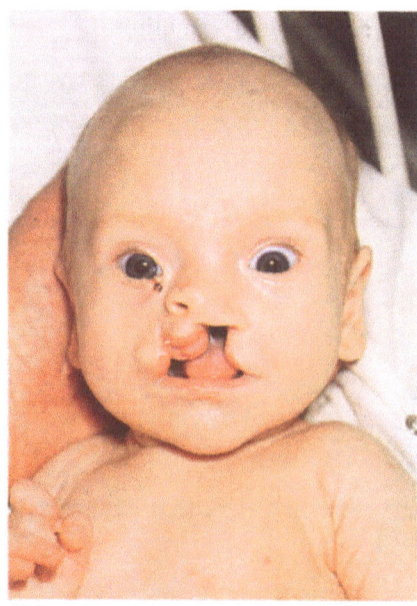

129 The right palpebral fissure is short and a hair-line coloboma in the lower lid has been repaired; false appearance of unilateral 'setting-sun' sign

Lateral deviation

This too may occur with minor neurological dysfunction [130], especially the hyperexcitability type. It remains to be seen how many cerebral lesions will be defined by non-invasive imaging [131] in neurological dysfunction and hemisyndromes in particular. One unusual child small for dates had congenital abnormalities and did not open her eyes until the age of 8 months. At first her eye opening was intermittent and was not full until 2 years [131A] but her eyes were always 'locked' to the right. The family intelligently had her gaze towards the left and at 6 years the eye movements were equilibrated (there was moderate optic atrophy). The underlying disorder proved to be partial trisomy-12 – CT scan at age 8 [131B].

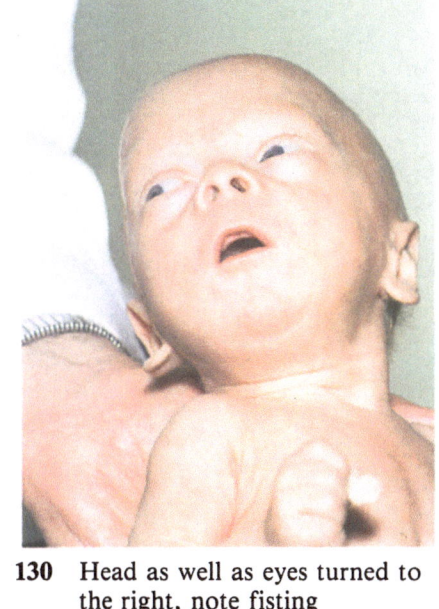

130 Head as well as eyes turned to the right, note fisting

Deviation upward/lateral

Two cases are illustrated here.

(1) One curious child showed upward deviation from birth, *sursumversion* for latinists, at 2 months this was still strong [132] and there was global developmental delay of obscure origin. At 6 months deviation was to the left [133] and air study showed asymmetrical ventricular dilatation [134] so this was taken to be gaze *contraversion* away from the more actively affected hemisphere.

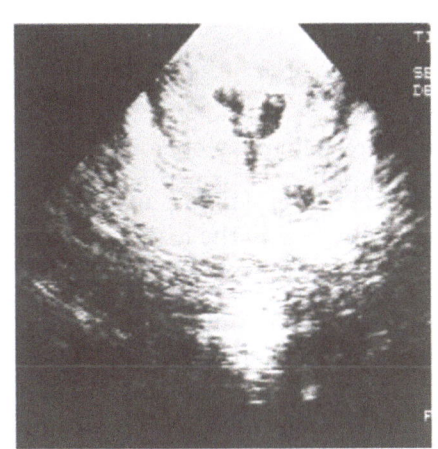

131 Parenchymal haemorrhage under the floor of the right lateral ventricle pushes it upwards

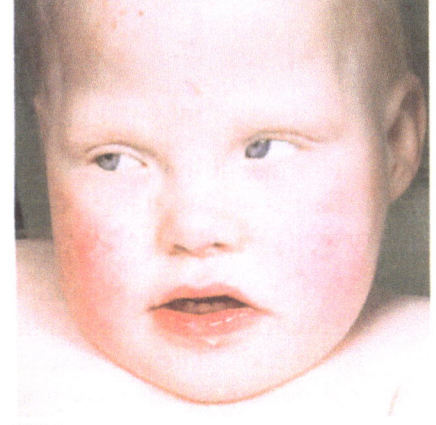

131A

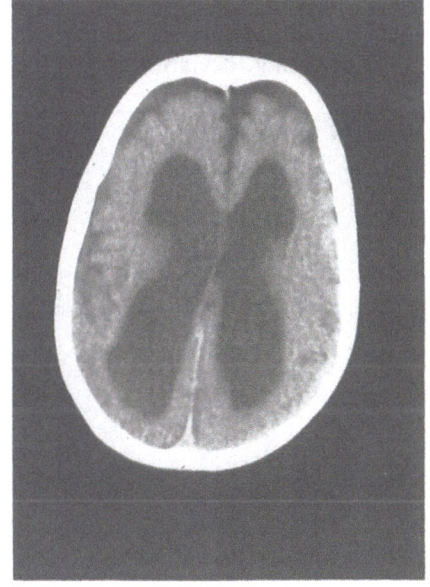

131B

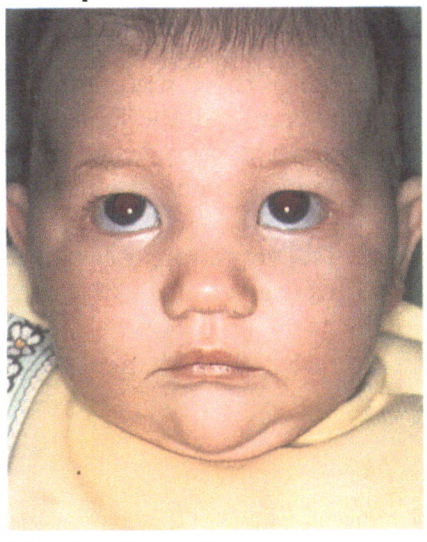

132 Age 2 months

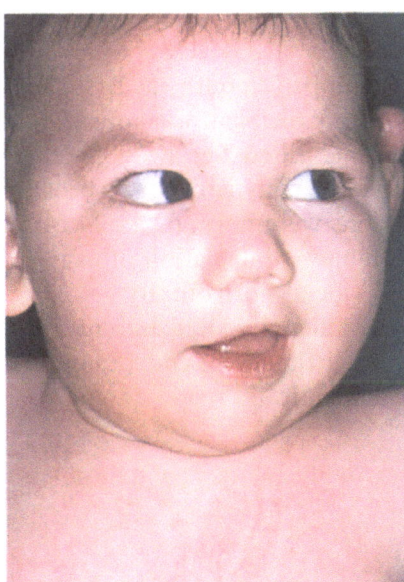

133 Age 6 months

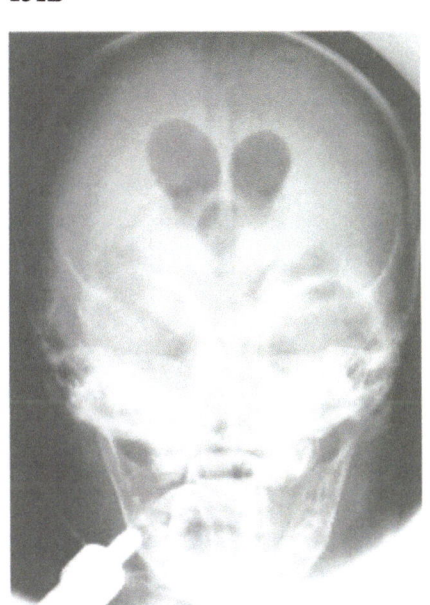

134 Age 6 months

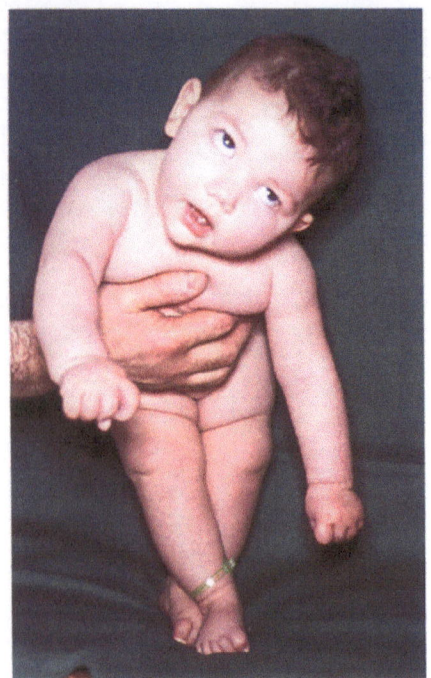

135 Poor head support, fisting, scissoring, deviation of eyes upwards and to left

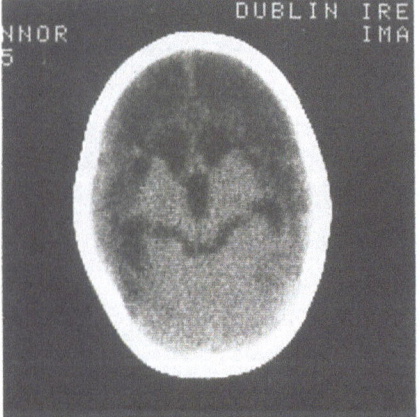

137 Extensive loss of cerebral tissue, but . . .

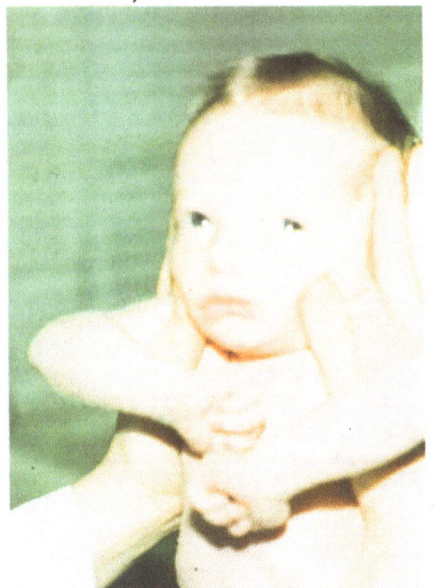

139 Age 2 weeks

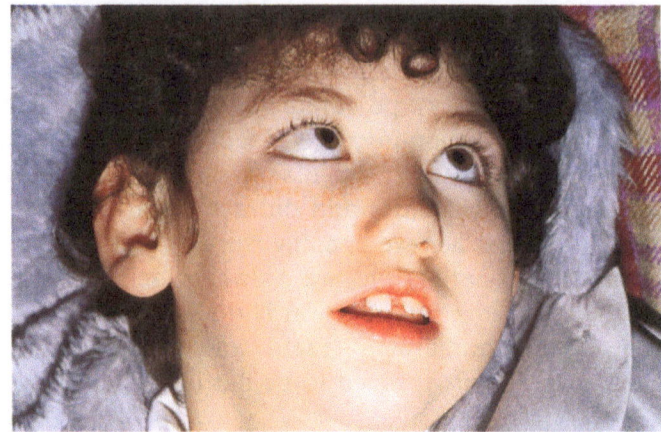

136 Ten years' eye deviation almost unchanged with . . .

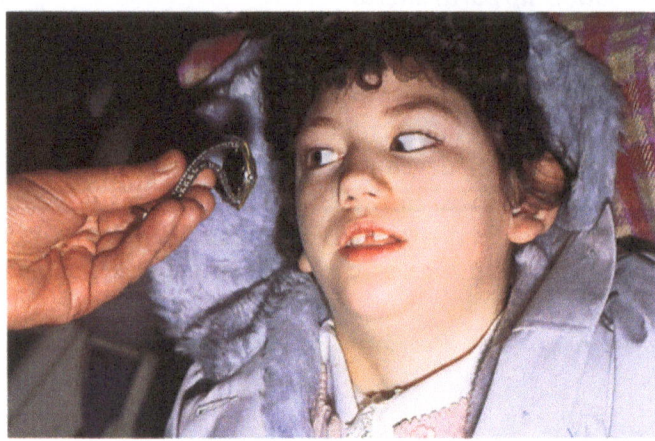

138 Her gaze is now led readily to the opposite extreme

Her condition was one of decerebration [135] and this has persisted to date [136] with a massive advance in the loss of cerebral tissue [137], although her gaze can be led to the extreme right [138].

(2) Another baby showed similar strong deviation only in response to the 'doll's eye' (upright) manoeuvre [139]; there was neurological dysfunction. The response faded imperceptibly over many months, routine inspections were normal, there is moderate developmental delay.

Deviation upward

A child of 8 months at first seemed to show 'gaze avoidance' [140] but the basic problem was upward gaze present from birth [141]; apparently she had tilted her head to correct her horizon. There was moderate generalized hypertonus, especially in the upper limbs. All special investigations were normal. At 2 years there is moderate developmental delay with upward deviation of gaze [142] but eye contact can be coaxed [143, 144] ahead horizontally.

Another child had extreme deviation [145, 146] very strongly sustained from birth; severe changes on CT scan [147] were associated with steady deterioration.

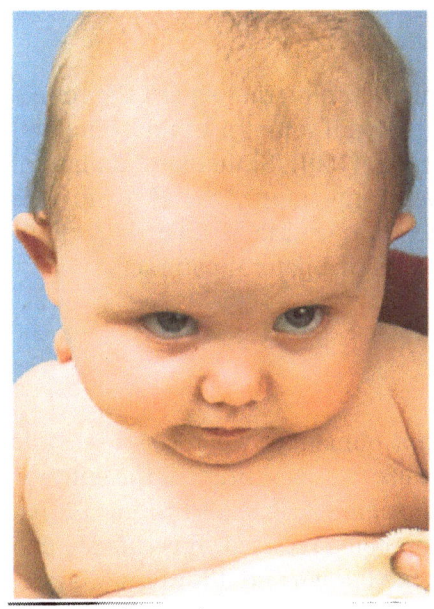

140 Age 8 months

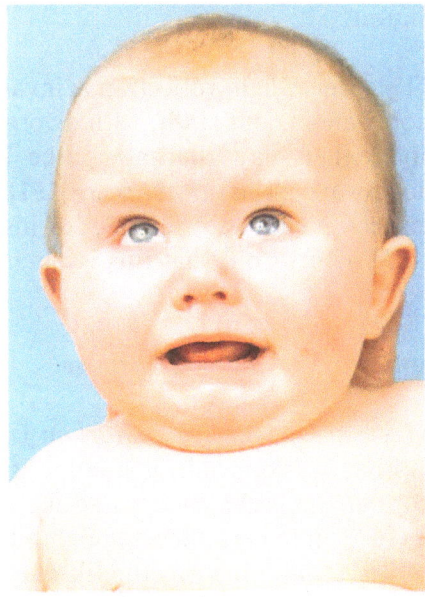

141 Age 2 months

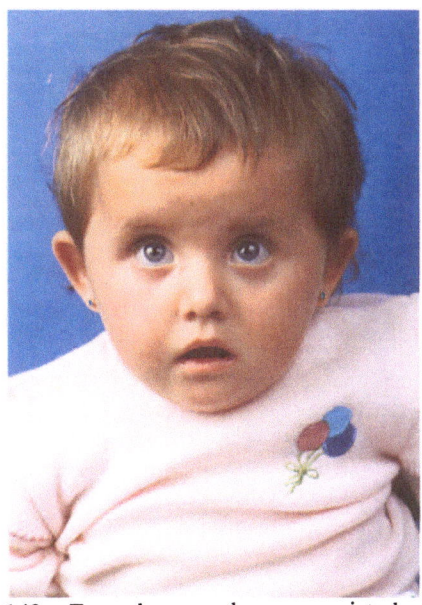

142 Forced upward gaze persists but it is stronger than before and . . .

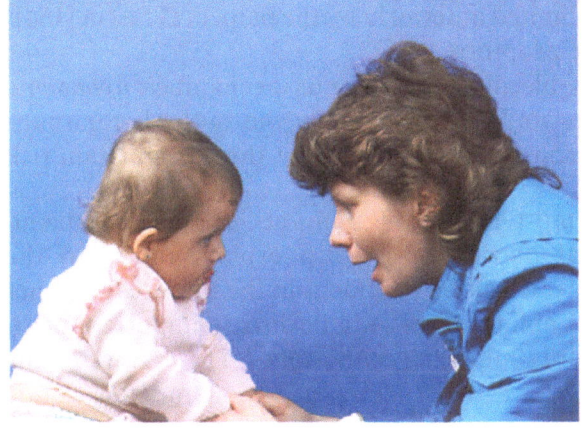

143 In play with the mother the head begins to come up . . .

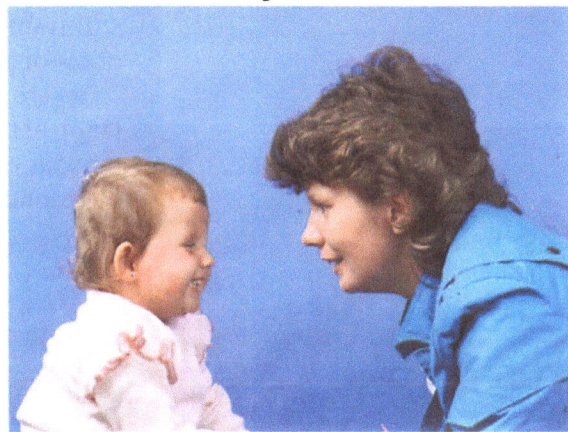

144 Until there is face-to-face confrontation

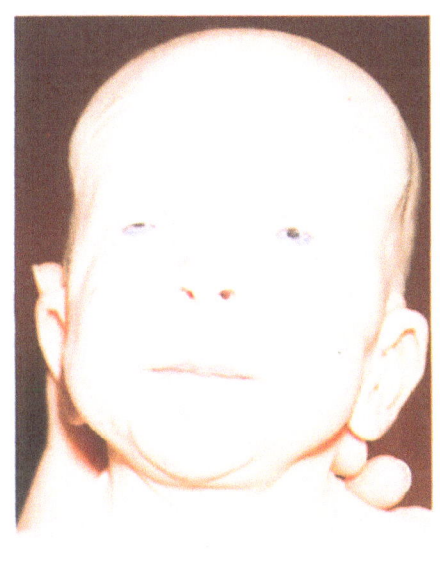

145 Aged 10 weeks

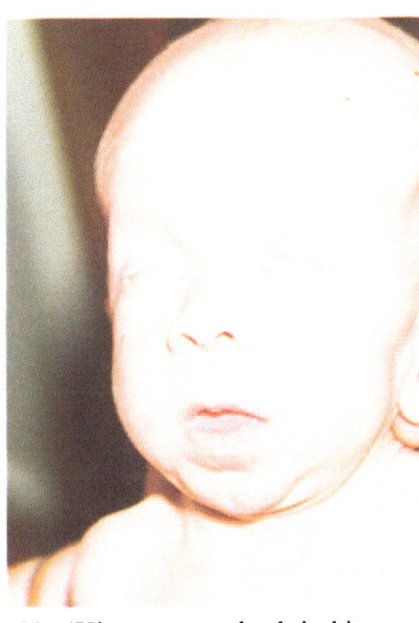

146 'His eyes went back in his head'

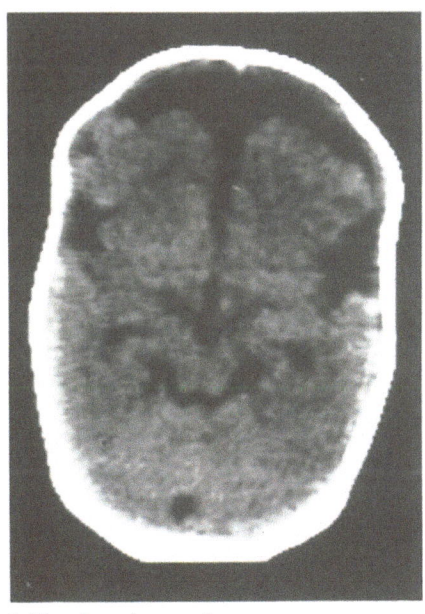

147 Age 4 months

Squint

The corneal light reflection is invaluable; with internal squint the reflection wanders out [148], with divergent external squint it wanders in [149] and either may alternate or be bilateral [150]. Sometimes unilateral downward deviation is seen [151]. With any squint, the eyes must be inspected with special care, for instance in one case of divergent squint [152] it turns out that this is the indicator of bilateral cataract.

Subconjunctival haemorrhage

This is truly the *pons asinorum*; I cannot remember when last a sensible mother overlooked it. It stands out because vessels rupture at the anterior part of the globe [see 4] and it shines bright red because room oxygen diffuses in to keep the haemoglobin from being reduced. It is ring-shaped because that is the way the fibres are tacked down and it is often bilateral because of the causative forces. In many cases there is a clue from signs of trauma round and about the lids [153].

Intraorbital bleeding is limited anteriorly by the palpebral fascia [154], occasionally there may be proptosis [155].

Severe trauma may cause bleeding into the anterior chamber: *hyphaema* [156] here due to forceps application. Happily the outlook for spontaneous early complete resolution is excellent, but there is a certain risk of secondary glaucoma.

The most important thing about finding subconjunctival haemorrhage is to explain things to the mother; she will be confident in the knowledge of her doctor's ability. It may not be disease-important but it is certainly humanely important ('The essence of the consultation is the explanation' – Sir James Spence). If anyone is so brash as to say 'that's nothing', our colleagues specialist in the psyche are quick to point out

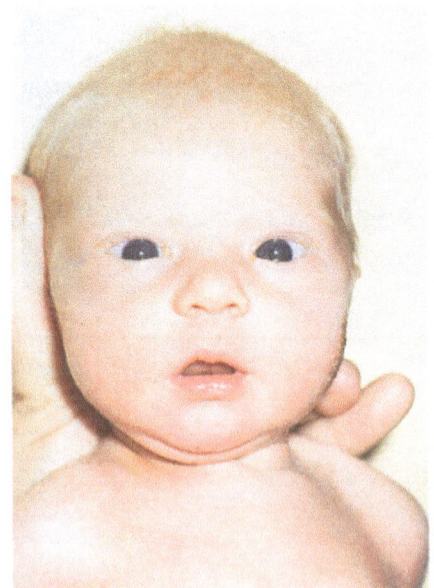

148

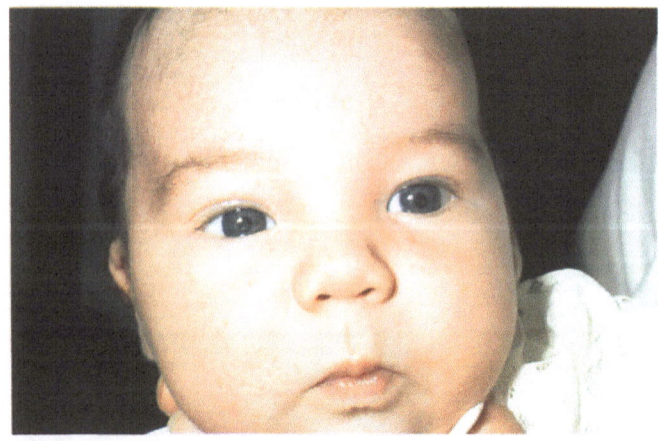

149

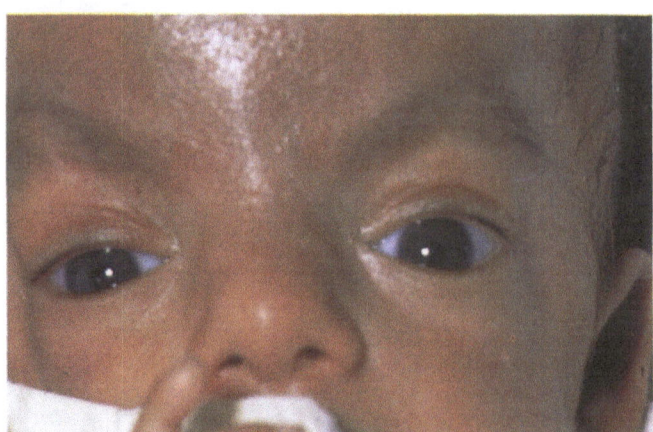

150   Note antimongolian slant

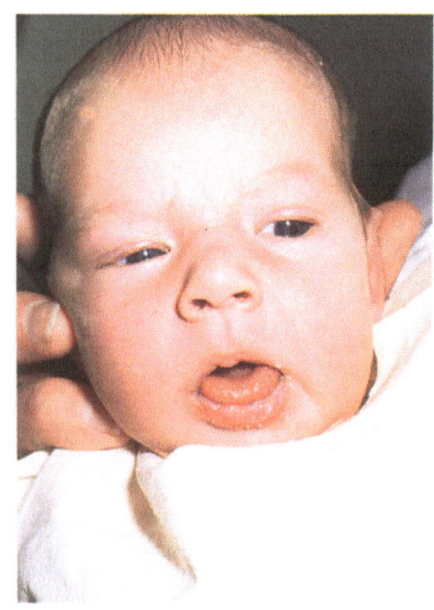

151

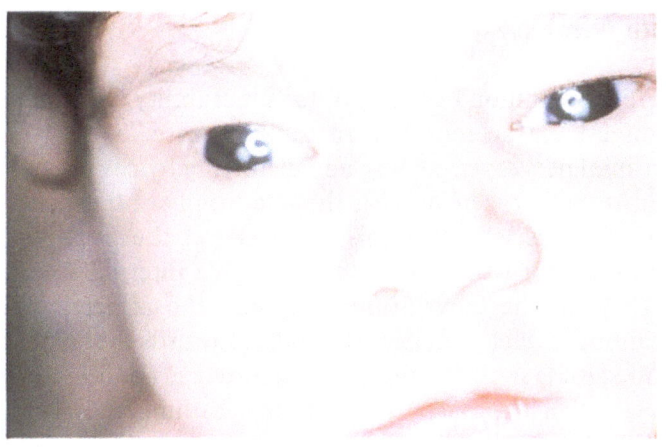

152

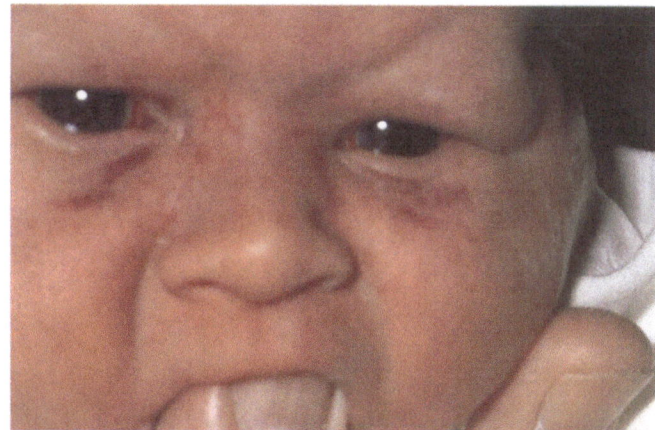

153

that that is the doctor speaking to himself. The clinician must remember the possible association of similar small haemorrhages [157] in sensitive danger areas. In the exceptional case massive intracerebral bleeding may occur [158]; in this instance the baby had a bleeding disorder.

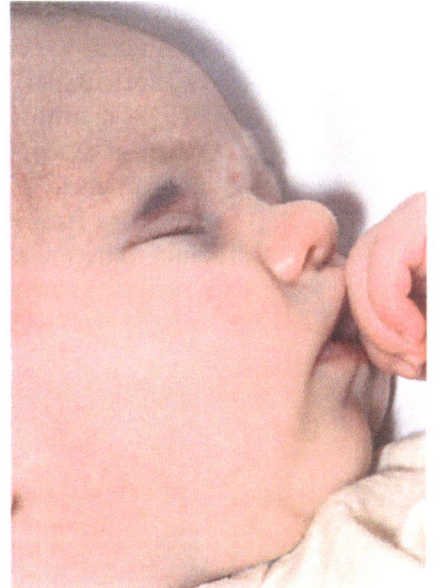

154

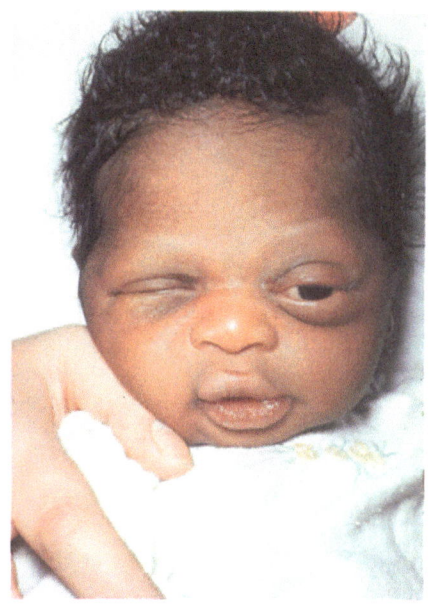

155

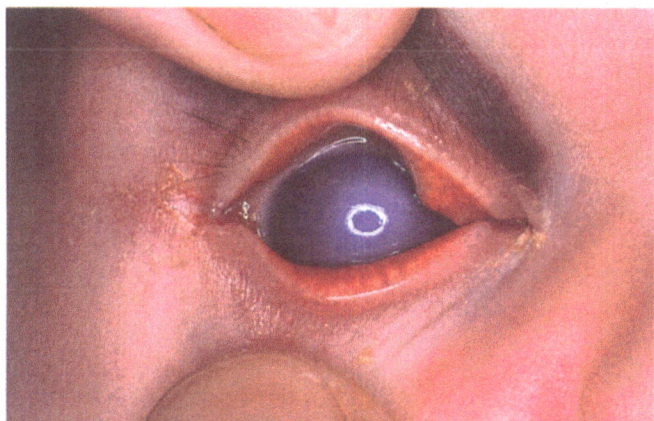

156 Serum and red cells may separate

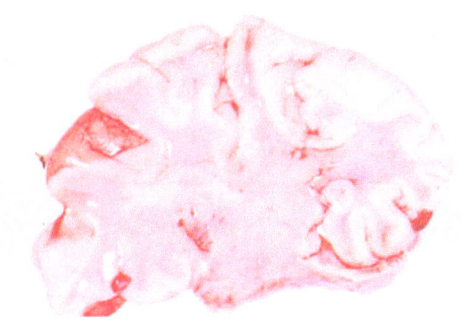

157

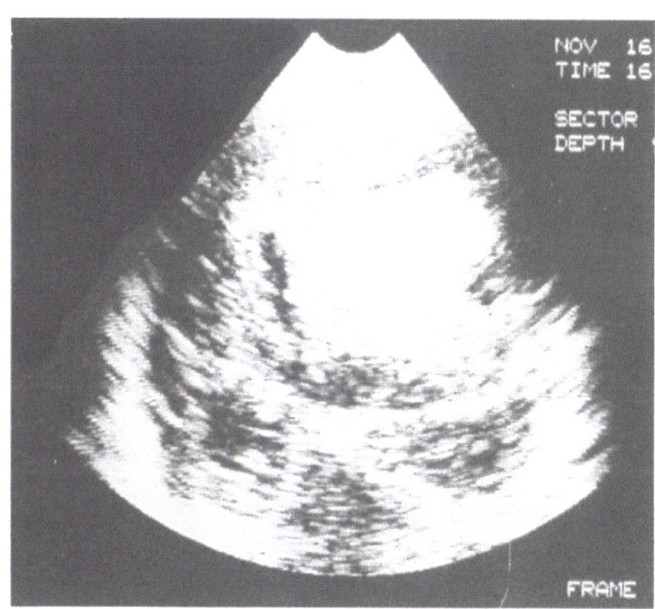

158 Large parenchymal haemorrhage right of centre

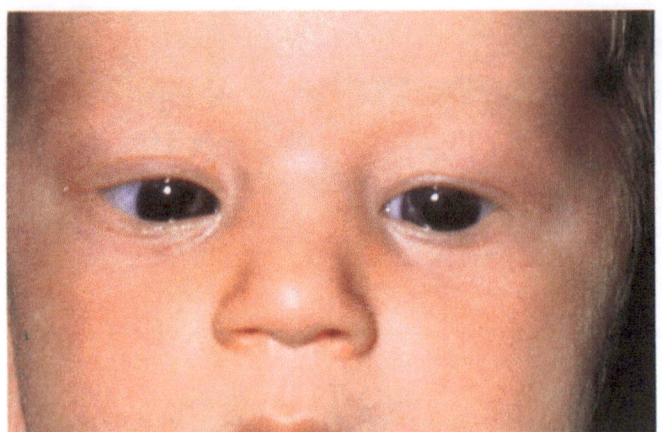

159 Right abducens palsy, neutral position. Internal squint at rest

6th Nerve palsy

This is common because of its vulnerability. It has the longest extracerebral intracranial course among the cranial nerves; stretching and distorting forces affect it most readily. The nerve is the sole supply of the lateral rectus muscle; when this is paralysed the opponent muscles turn the eye inwards to give internal squint [159]. In the labyrinthine response the affected eye cannot abduct, i.e., turn (laterally) towards the leading side [160], so the squint is exaggerated as the other eye *does* turn (medially) towards the leading side [161]. With bilateral 6th nerve palsy there is *convergent* squint [162] as both eyes turn inwards; trauma can cause this, but here it is due to the *Möbius syndrome* of nuclear agenesis; something peculiar like this might be anticipated from the story of easy spontaneous delivery. In this instance [163], the bilateral 6th nerve palsy is associated with left 7th nerve lower motor neuron palsy (the eye could not close) and there is epiphora from malformation of the left nasolacrimal duct. There was associated hypoplasia and deformity [164] of some digits of the left hand. The degree of micrognathos is typical.

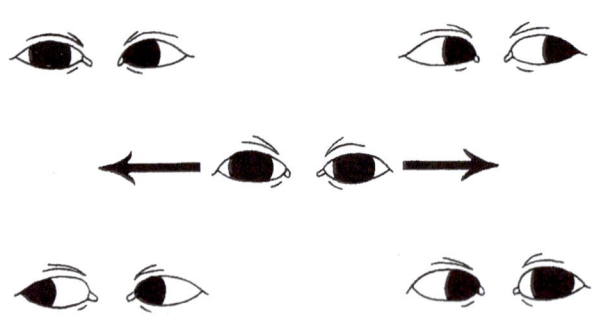

160 Abducens (6th nerve) palsy: top right-sided, bottom left-sided. The eyes at rest are shown straight

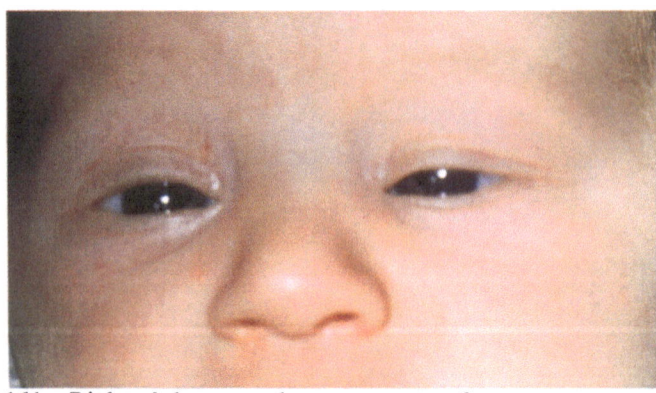

161 Right abducens palsy at extreme of movement to the baby's right in labyrinthine reflex

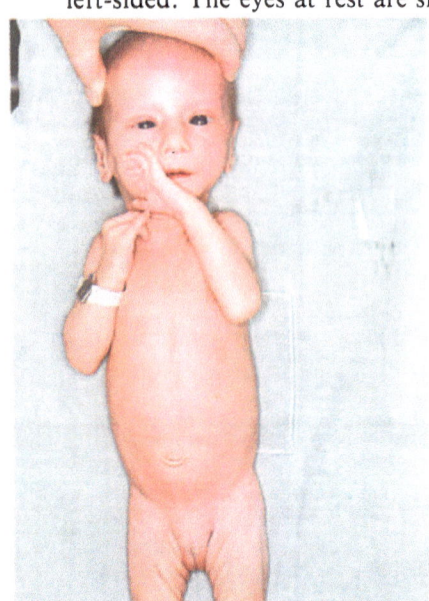

162

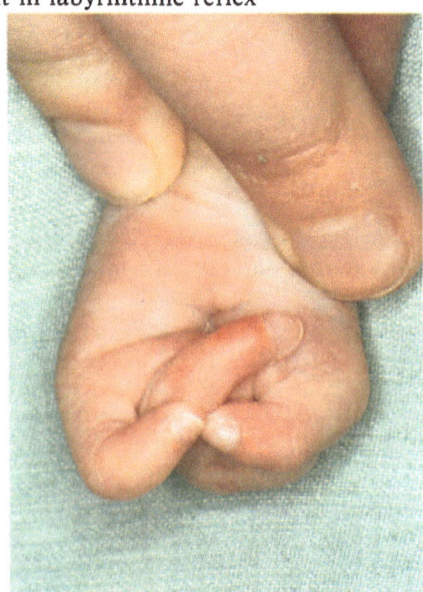

163 Bilateral 7th palsy, left greater than right

164

Other

This category covers anything further that may be found, a bonus beyond our irreducible minimum. For a change, it is usually something structural that is seen and it will come more readily to the notice of the doctor who knows the method of wide eye-opening. There may be other stigmas to be found, but the whole situation cannot be understood until we always see each baby as a combination of his inheritance (genetic) and his life-experience to date (events of pregnancy and delivery). This is essential to understanding the patient, otherwise the routine work of the nursery becomes very dull and unrewarding.

Retinoscopy

Retinoscopy is mandatory when there is a significant clinical finding, before consulting the ophthalmologist. It was a salutary albeit exceptional lesson to glimpse naked-eye [165] something unremarked on referral. The disc [166] and the macula are of prime importance [167]. At the macula the cherry-red spot is legendary in Tay–Sachs lipidosis of Ashkenazi Jews, so this spot, in a gentile child [168], probably means the similar Sandhoff disease. This case was found through neurological dysfunction/non-risk performance in the nursery. However, in another unusual instance the

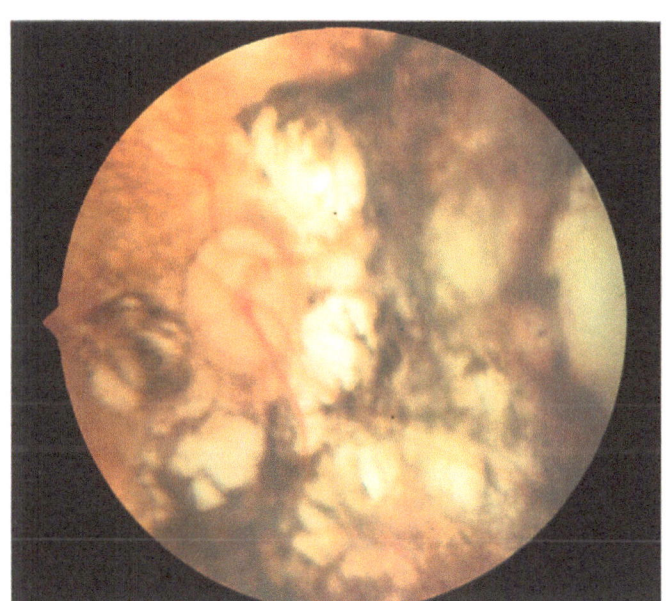

165   Colobomas, *cf*.401

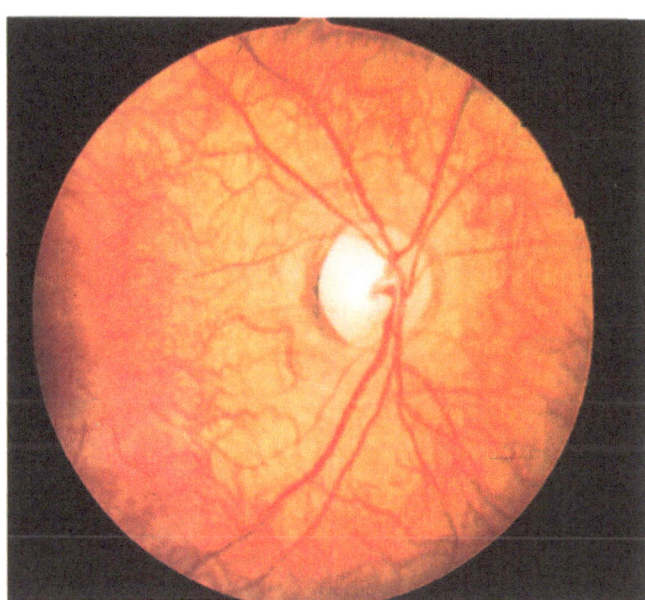

166   Optic atrophy. The 'retinal' vessels are prominent; mainly choroidal, showing through thin choroid

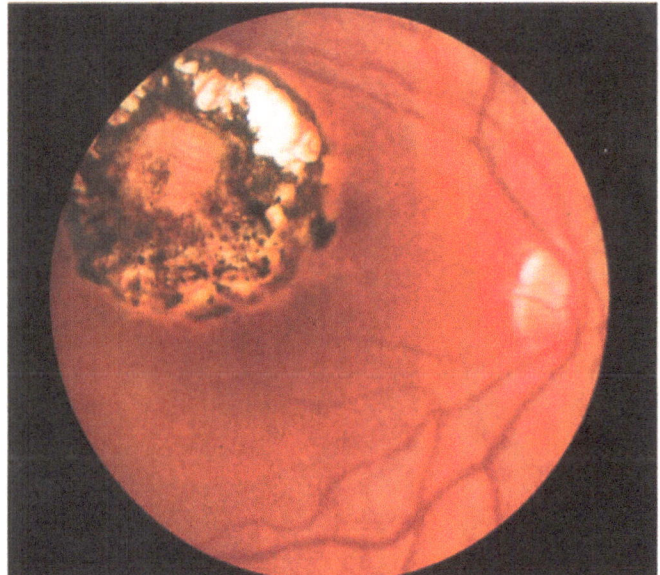

167   Chorioretinitis of toxoplasmosis

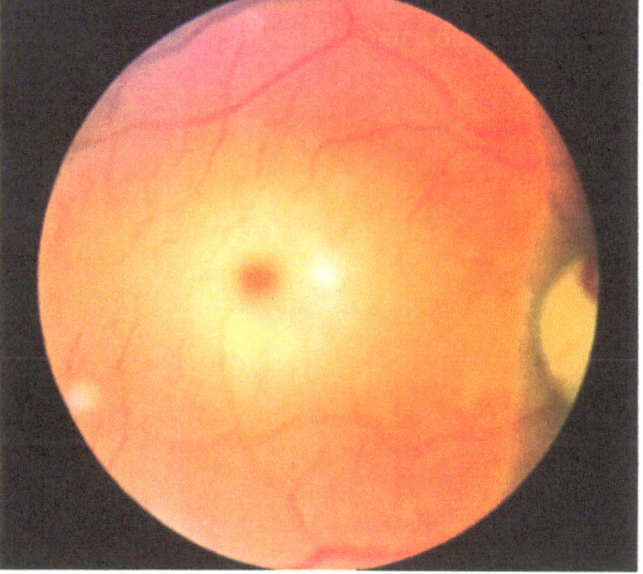

168   Age 4 weeks

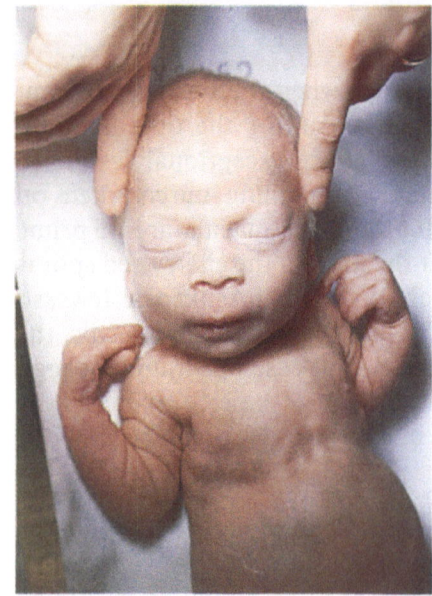

169

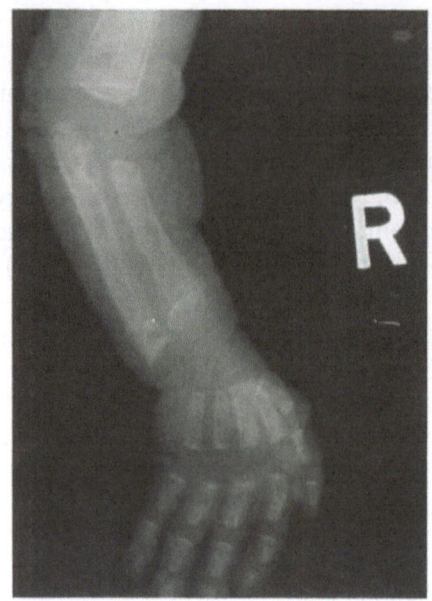

170

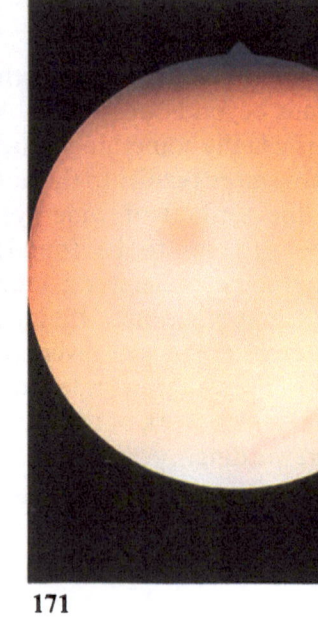

171

phenotype can point to possible cherry-red spot: the Caffey pseudo-Hurler GM$_1$ gangliosidosis Type I [169], the appearance is typical and on X-ray the bones are 'cloaked' [170], 50% have the cherry-red spot [171] with less than the awful brilliance of Tay–Sachs or Sandhoff. The pseudo-Hurler is of recessive inheritance [172, 173].

In a baby with Hurler's disease the expected optic atrophy was found [174], together with an illusion of 'cherry-red spot': the retinal pallor normal for age had simply brightened the normal macular light reflex. Hurler does not develop a cherry-red spot. A baby with rotatory nystagmus had hypoplastic optic disks with retinal atrophy [175], no named diagnosis to date.

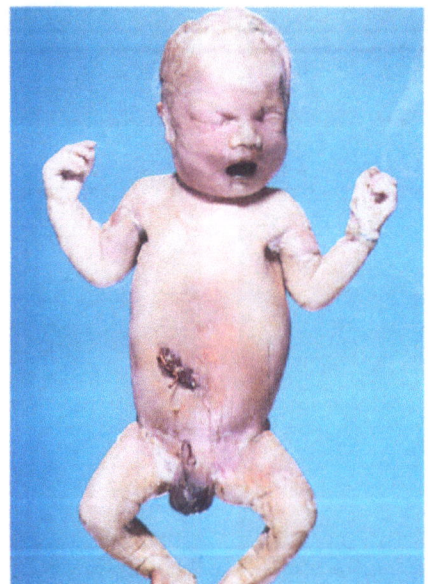

172

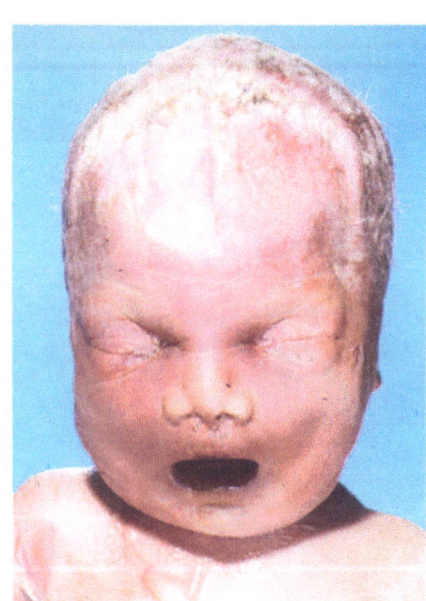

173

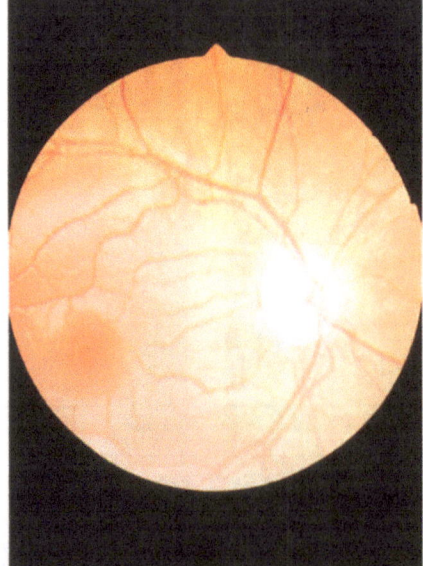

174   Age 16 months

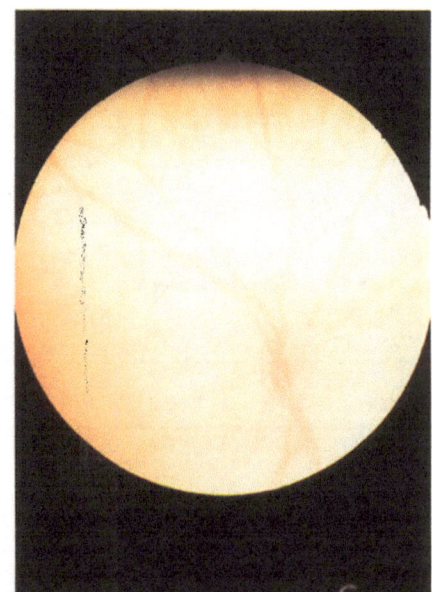

175

PART II

FURTHER OCCASIONAL FINDINGS

George Herbert, 5th Earl of Carnarvon: '*Can you see anything?*'
Howard Carter: '*Yes, wonderful things.*'
(Tomb of Tutankhamun, 1922)

The feasibility of the basic proposal is honoured by keeping the diagnostic illustrations to the neonatal period, with a couple of inevitable exceptions.

An attempt is made to impose order by starting at the centre (*pupil*) and looking stepwise to the periphery (*surrounding territory*).

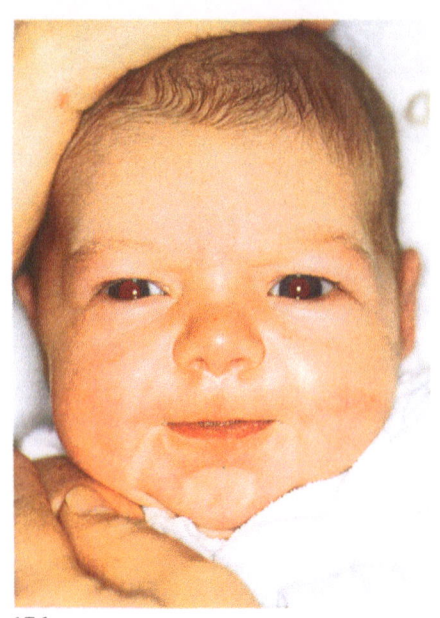

176

THE PUPIL

The normal pupil shows the *red reflex* [176]. This means that the tissues are clear all the way back to the retina and the light rays shone in through the pupil are reflected back off the retina. Photographers hate to produce it inadvertently [see 366] – it counts as an error of technique caused by holding the flash parallel to the depths of the fundus.

The pupil may show white (leukokoria) because of dense fibrous material behind it. This is usually cataract [177]; this rubella baby had contralateral microphthalmos [178], she succumbed to heart disease. Rubella was always suspected if cataracts [179] were associated with a purpuric rash like this one, or one that was infiltrative [180]. The optic fundi might show

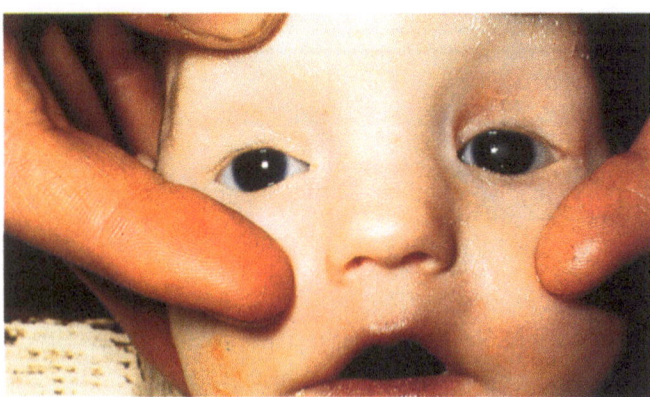

177

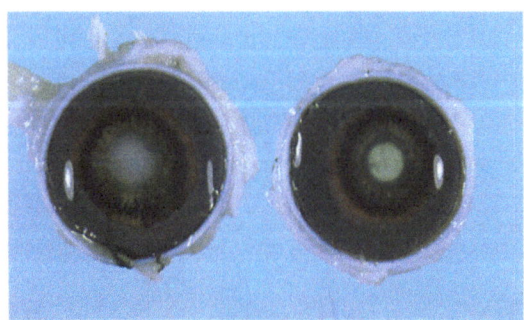

178

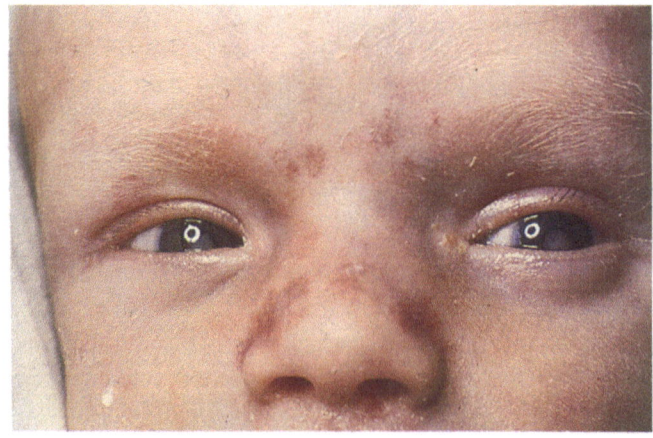

179

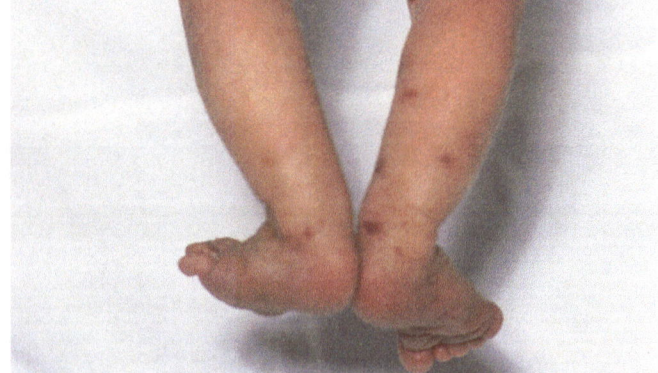

180

the typical 'pepper-and-salt' retinopathy [181]. With purpura, there is usually thrombocytopenia and femoral X-ray may show streaky linear decalcification from osteitis [182], the 'celery stalk' appearance [see also 107, 227]. Prima facie evidence along these lines makes barrier nursing imperative to protect susceptible females; the babies are virus excretors. The bones soon heal, the purpura fades [183] and the X-rays return to normal. Because the rubella virus has a continuing noxious effect on the inner ear it is important to anticipate possible deafness [184] by following these children through to school entry, until the full range of hearing can be tested and they are shown to be speaking normally.

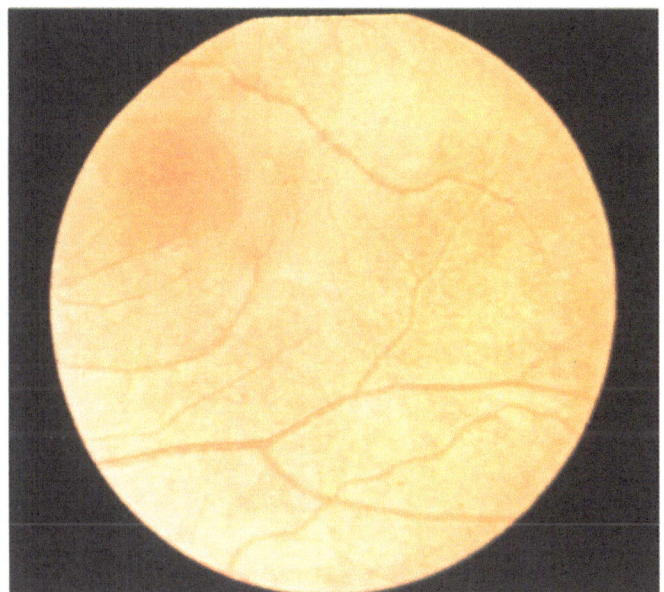

181   'Pepper and salt' retinitis

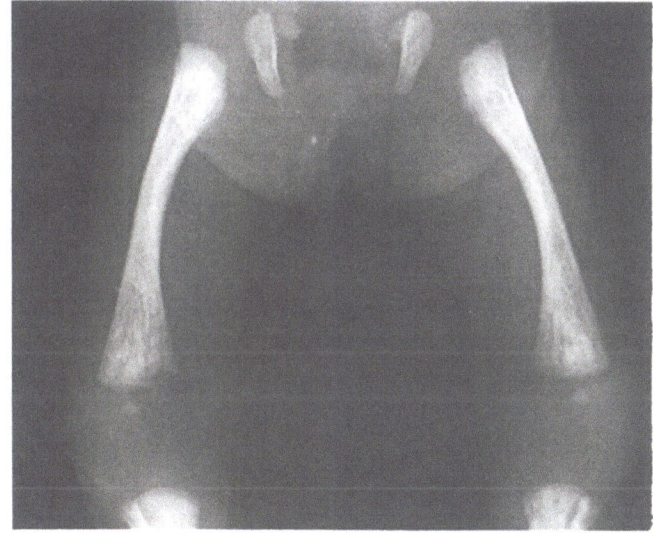

182

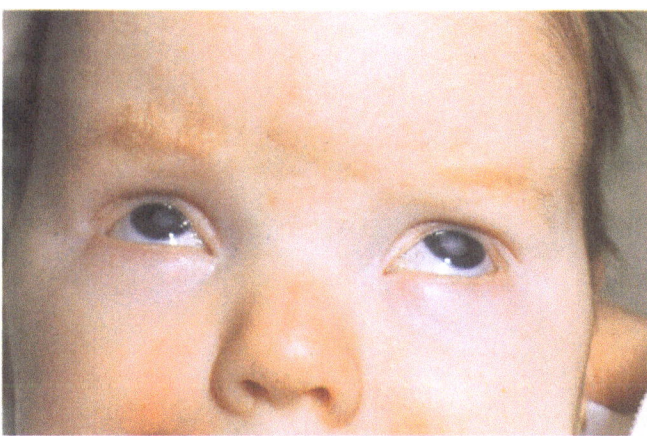

183   Age 8 weeks, note right eye smaller

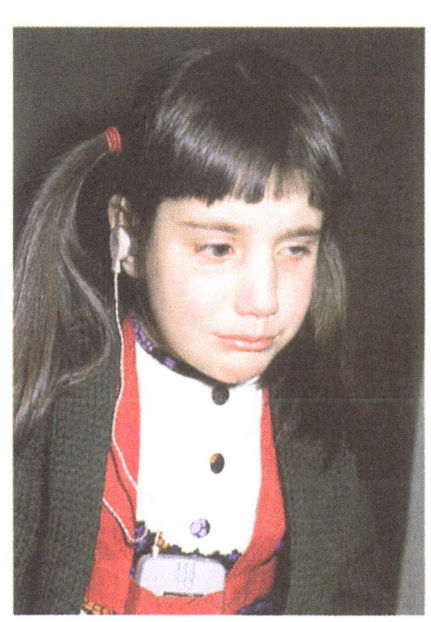

184

Galactosaemia [185] and similar inherited metabolic disorders cause the most urgent cataract of all; this child did not survive because liver damage was so severe. At the other end of the spectrum, some cataracts [186] may be left alone if they admit sufficient light round the periphery to counterbalance the hazard of surgery [see 13].

Some other possible causes of leukokoria are retinal dysplasia, retinoblastoma, retrolental fibroplasia, incontinentia pigmenti 'pseudoglioma', primary vitreous hyperplasia . . . these rarities have one other feature in common: they require the opinion of an ophthalmologist, *statim*.

Lens dislocation

This might be seen if there is a diagnosis of homocystinuria [187] by screening or from the story of an affected sibling; here the displacement is appropriately *downwards* and the child is aged 4; to date the youngest age recorded is 2 years. It might also be seen in Marfan's syndrome [188] if the clinician is astute – usually the family history is the tip-off; in this case we did not find the expected *upwards* displacement, all we saw was the rather blue sclerotics typical of this condition.

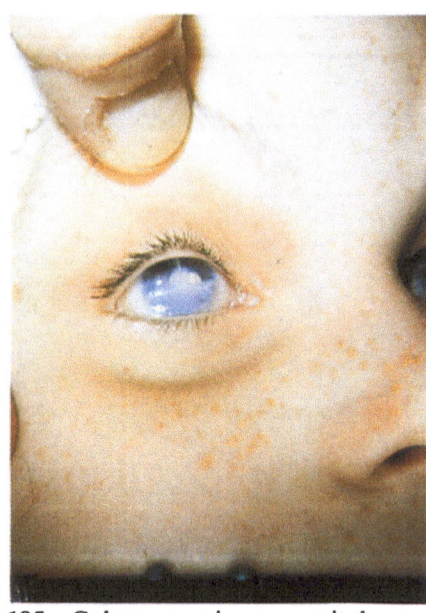

185   Galactosaemia, congenital cataracts

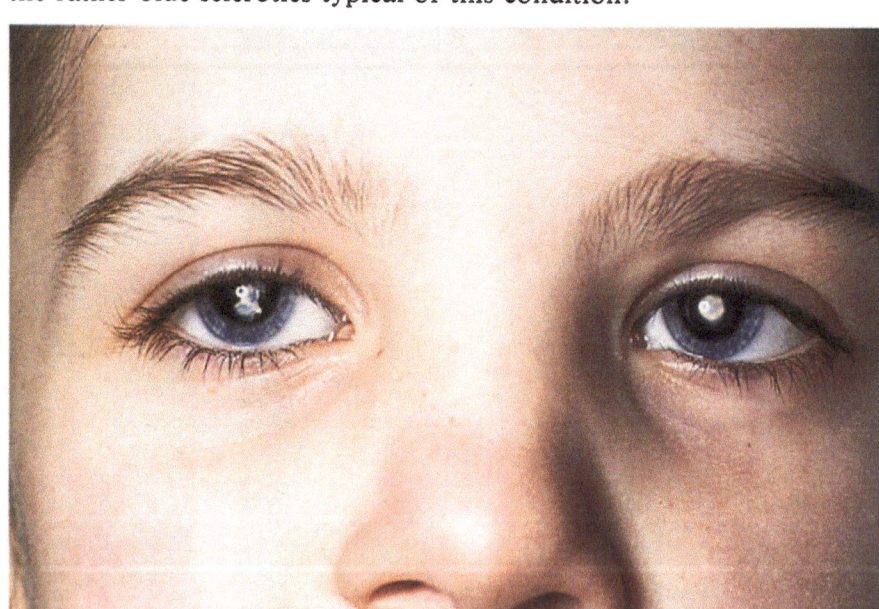

186

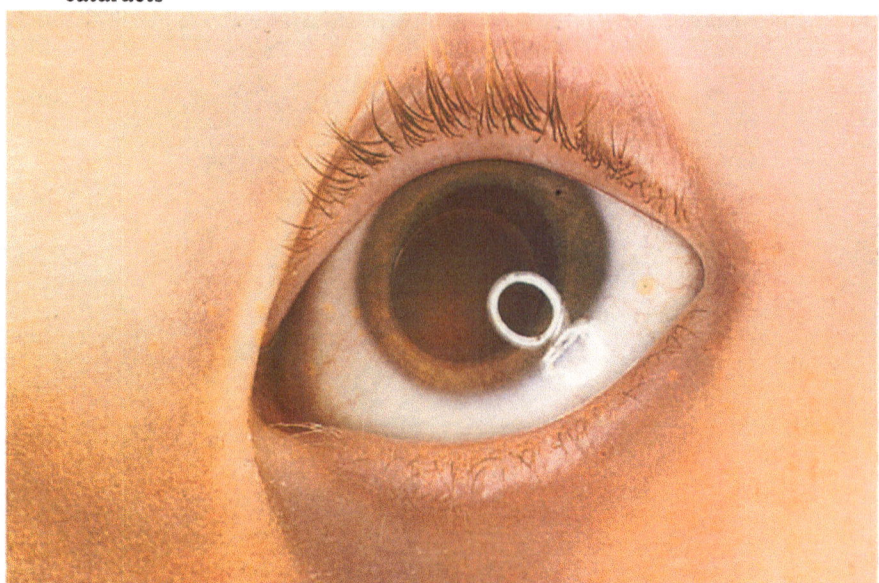

187   Suspensory ligament of lens is stretched

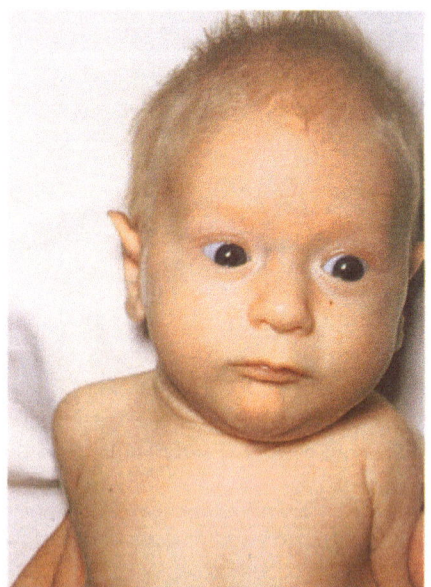

188

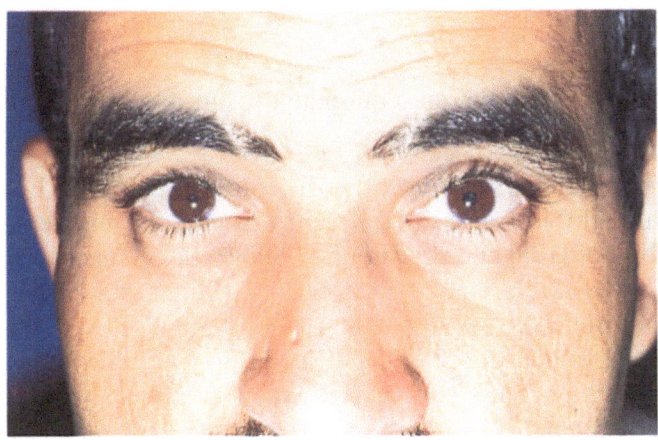

189 Associated anosmia

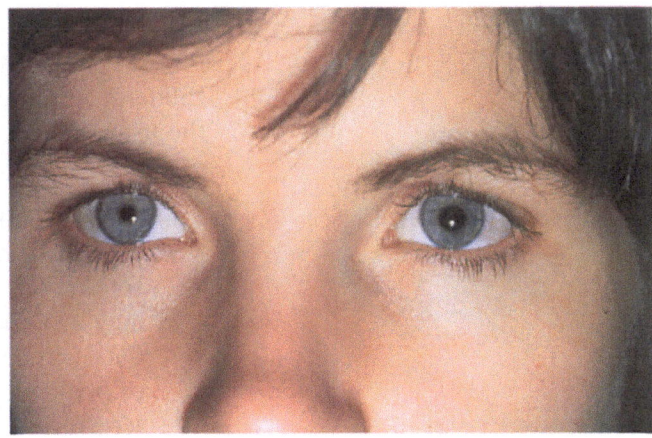

190 The unequal pupils probably present from birth, asymptomatic and no further diagnosis

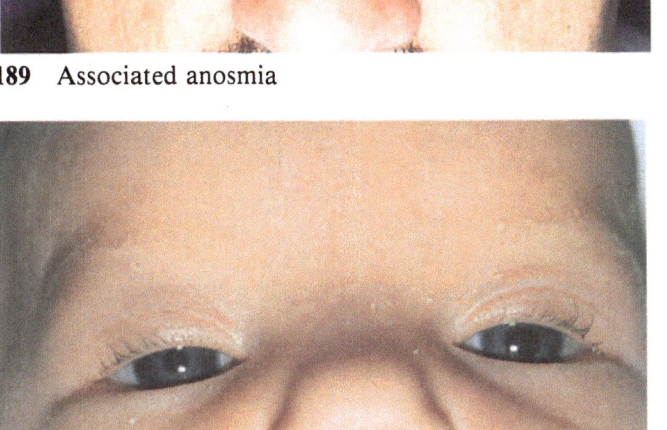

191

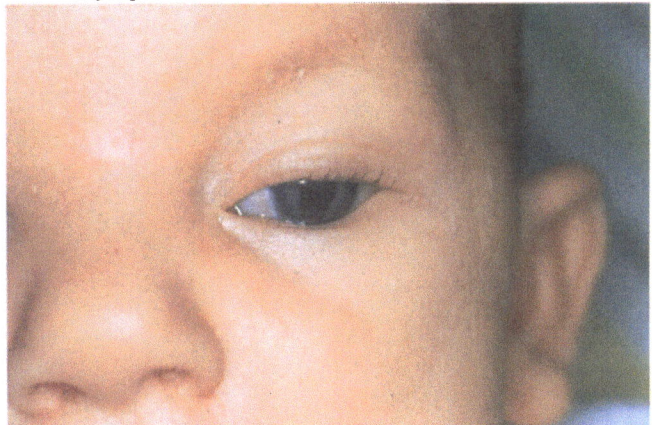

192 Coloboma revealed

Unequal pupils

Unequal pupils (anisocoria) discovered in infancy may well prove to be examples of Adie's tonic pupil, while others remain unexplained: [189] a postgraduate who also has anosmia, [190] a member of the nursing staff. When 'unequal pupils' are found unexpectedly [191], this merits close inspection which may reveal [192] an optical illusion, literally. This pitfall is not exclusive to the newborn period [193, 194].

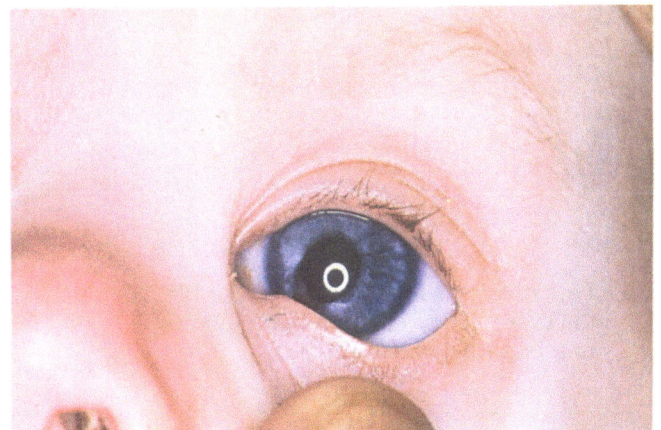

193

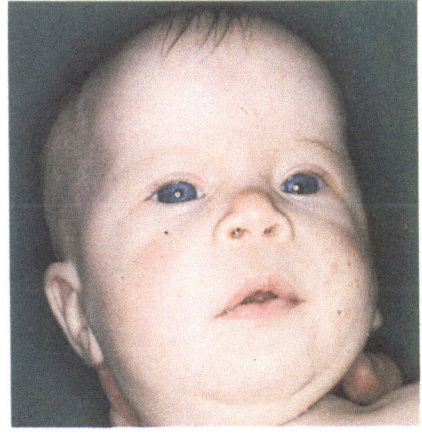

194

THE IRIS

Bilateral colour change is the commonest anomaly; forms of albinism are the usual cause.

(1) In classical *oculocutaneous albinism* the iris colour is pale blue but reddish-pink as light is transmitted freely through the pigment-deficient membranes [195] and the pupillary light reflex is an orange colour; the hair and skin are affected as well. The light hair colour may at first go unremarked in Caucasians, but it is vivid from the outset in babies of dark racial pigmentation [196]. The inheritance of oculocutaneous albinism is simple autosomal recessive [197, and see 96].

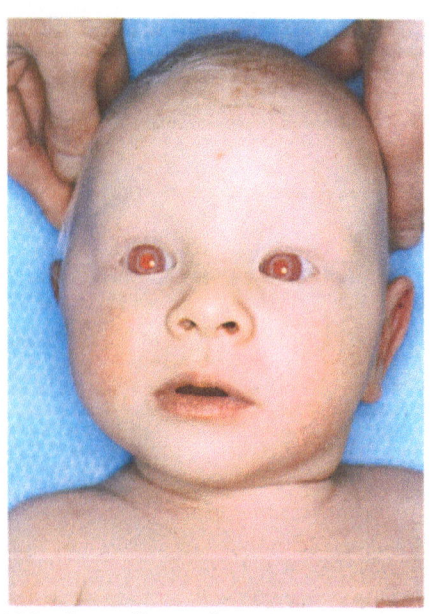

195 Late diagnosis at 3 months, the eyes were screwed up tight in a brightly-lighted nursery

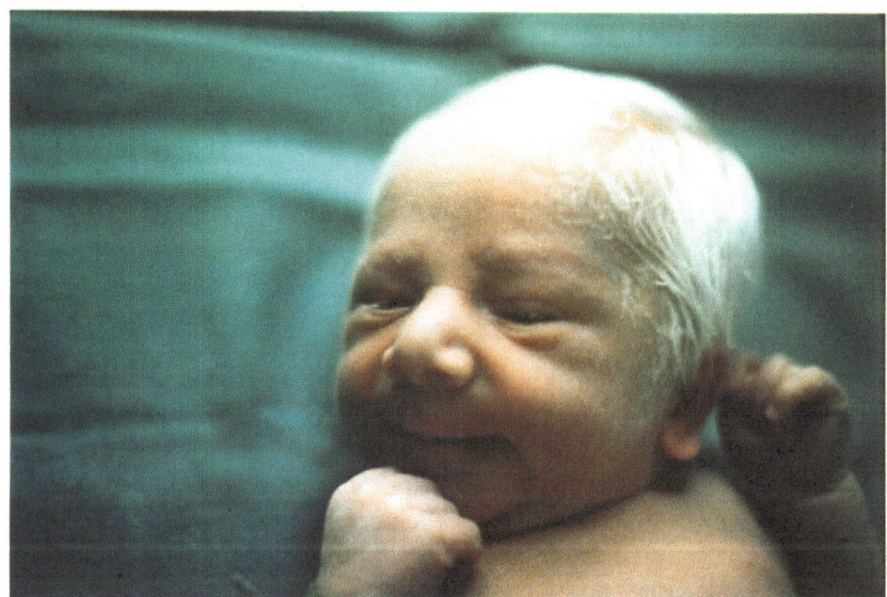

196 Arab baby

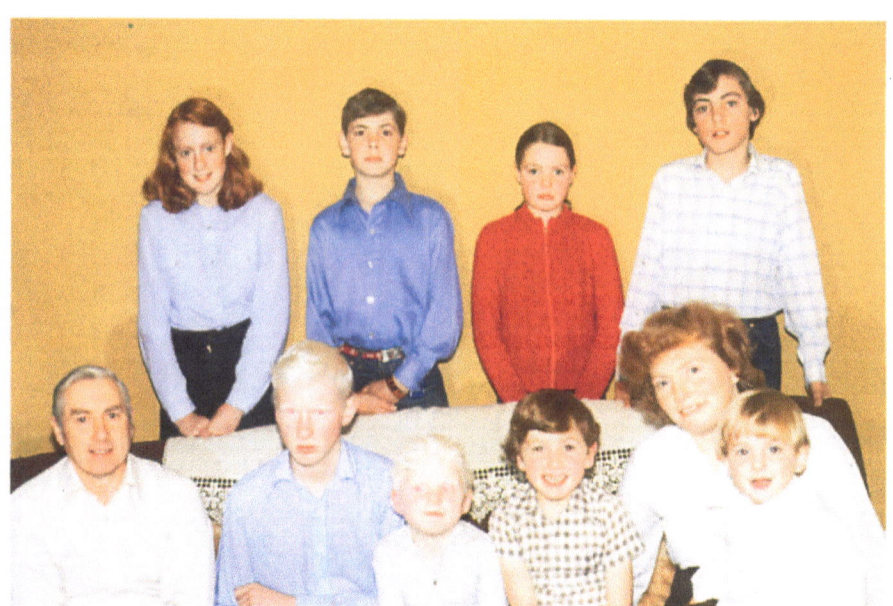

197 Practical clinical genetics in a typical happy Irish family

(2) In *ocular albinism* [198] the deficiency of pigment is confined to the iris and choroid. It is celebrated as one of the few eye defects that can be sex-linked recessive (Nettleship and Falls disorder: female carriers show a mosaic pattern fundus), but since this patient is female, hers is the alternative autosomal recessive condition; it is as severe as that of affected males and the obligate carriers have normal fundi.

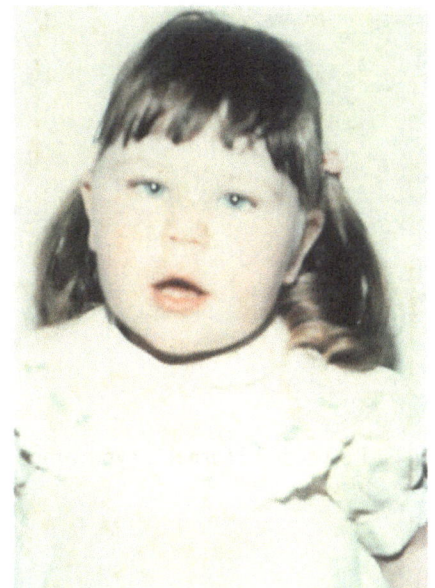

198

The iris colour is a striking pale blue [199] in a percentage of males [200] with the *fragile X mental deficiency syndrome* [201]. After puberty their enlarged testes and macrosomia are evident [202].

Bright blue irises occur in association with partial albinism or its opposite, partial melanism [203].

Heterochromia iris is a mixture of colours, and its classification is facilitated by borrowing terminology from the world of true hermaphroditism, viz., lateral, unilateral and bilateral heterochromia. For brown–blue this means Br + Bl (lateral), Br/Bl + Br or Bl (unilateral), Br/Bl + Br/Bl (bilateral).

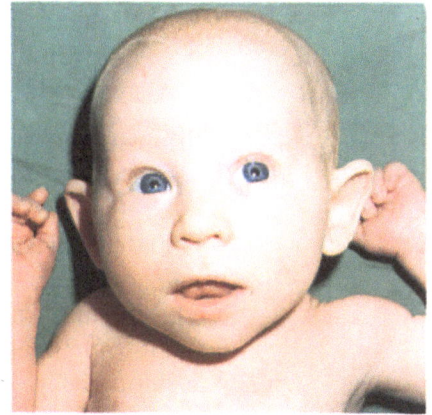

199 Age 3 months, neurological query eye colour and jug ears . . .

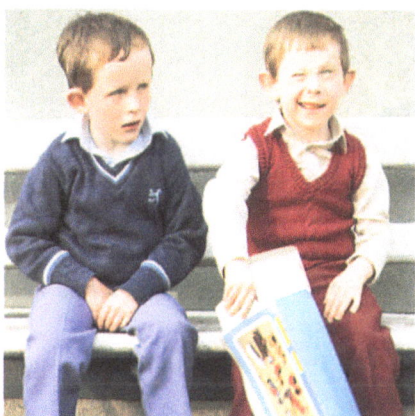

200 Led to brothers, age 8 years (left), 6 years (right)

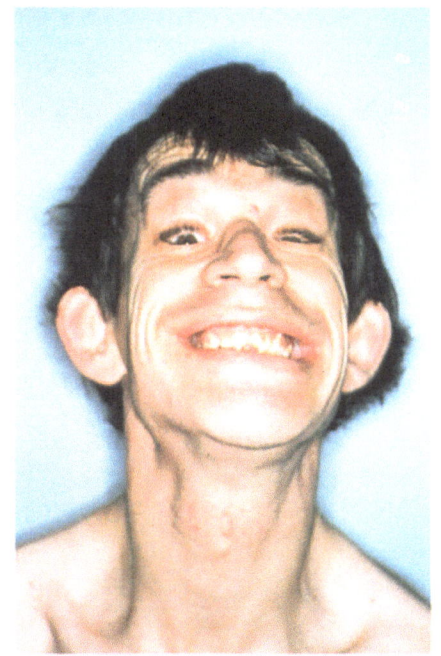

201 Brown-eyed patient

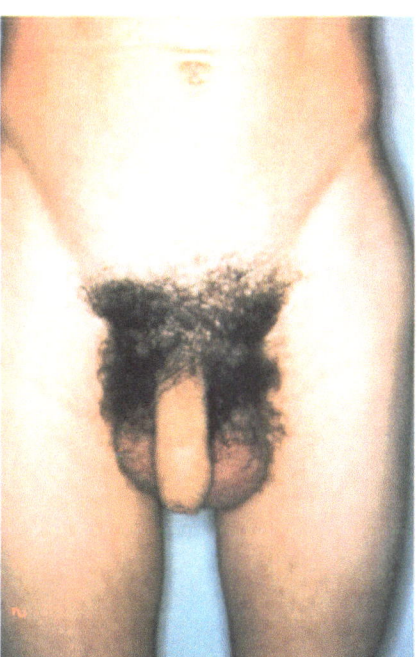

202

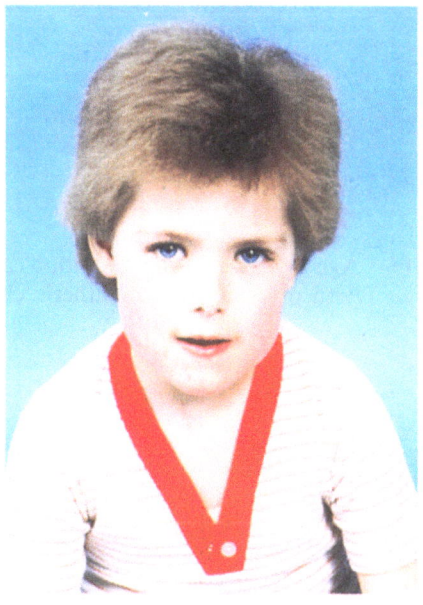

203

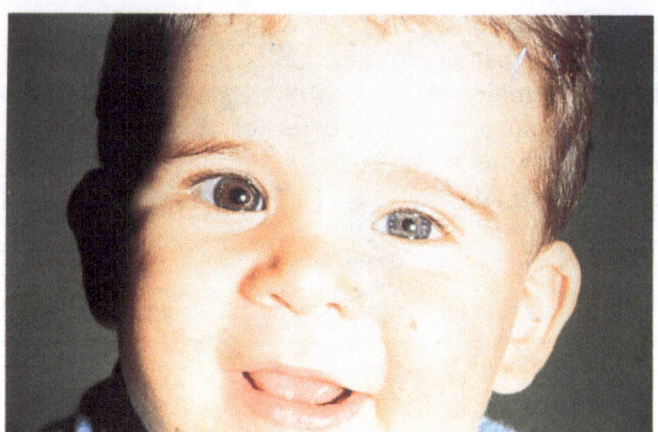

204　Left-sided Horner's syndrome

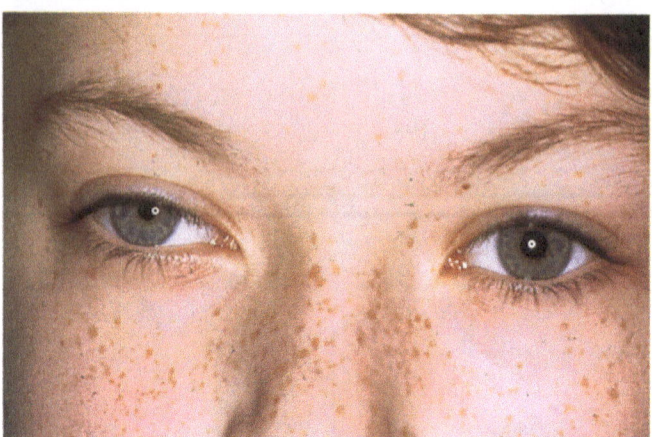

205　Spitz–Holter valve inserted at 6 weeks

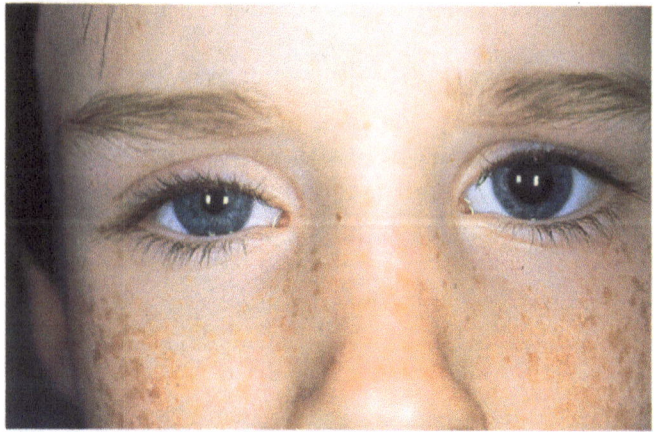

206　Age 4 years, Ewing's tumour causing rib destruction with pressure on sympathetic chain

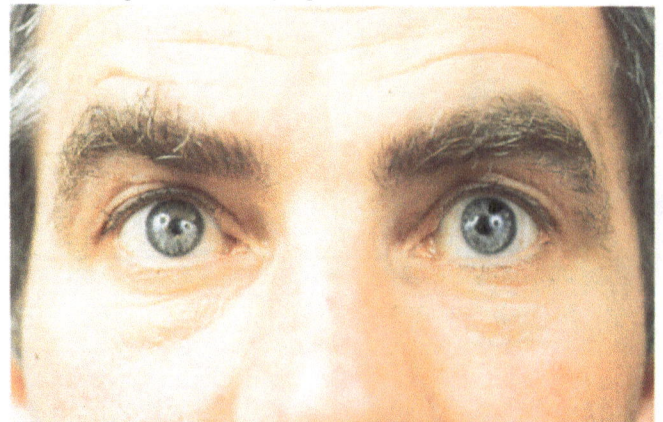

207　Note iridectomy scar

Lateral heterochromia (eyes of different colour):

Notorious

(i)　*Waardenburg's syndrome* [see 333].

(ii)　*Horner's syndrome* due to sympathetic nerve damage in early life interferes with secondary pigmentation of the iris [204, 205]. Since secondary pigmentation is completed by 2 years, another young Horner's should not have heterochromia [206]; his lesion arose at 4 years.

(iii)　*Fuchs' heterochromic cyclitis* [207] is a form of degeneration or atrophy of the iris with glaucoma and/or cataract; this man's heterochromia was remarked at age 18. Some patients have cervical rib.

Modest

(i)　'Casual' association following the rule that malformations tend to be multiple: this boy has cystic kidneys [208].

(ii)　Isolated heterochromia as an innocent stigma.

Unilateral heterochromia (different colours in the eye)

This is usually a small random splash of colour [18, 19] but it sometimes seems more 'organized' in a segmental fashion [209]. An unusual but well-known change is the *Lisch nodule* [210] of von Recklinghausen's disease. This last has a certain potential for malignant change, the others to a much lesser extent.

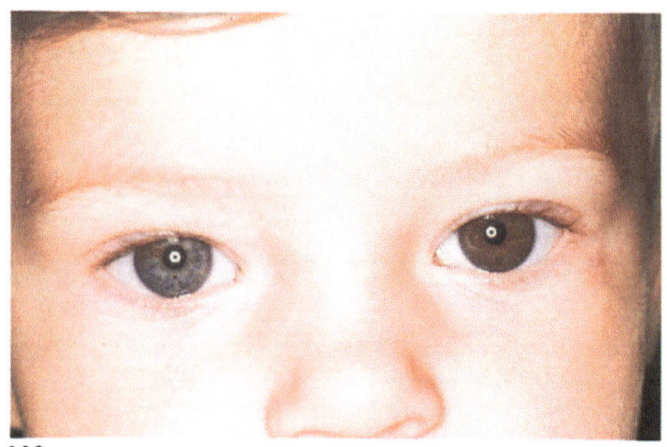

208

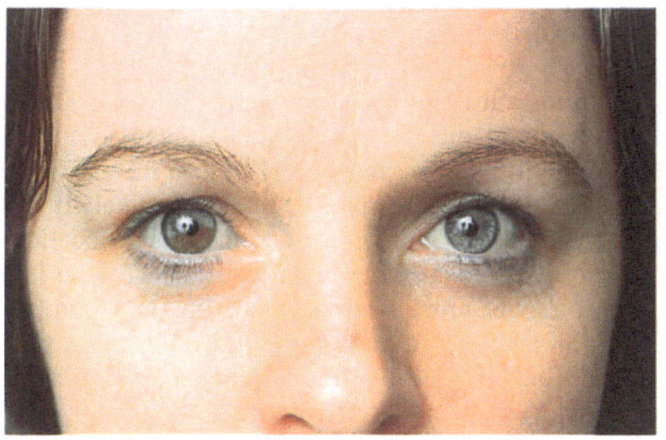

209 Segmental heterochromia

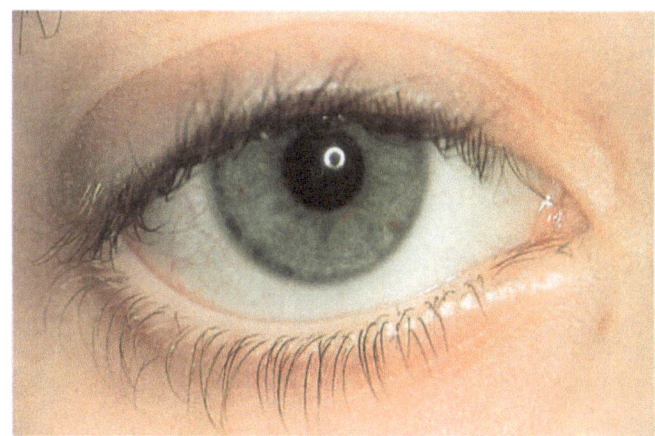

210 Age 6 years, small dense nodules

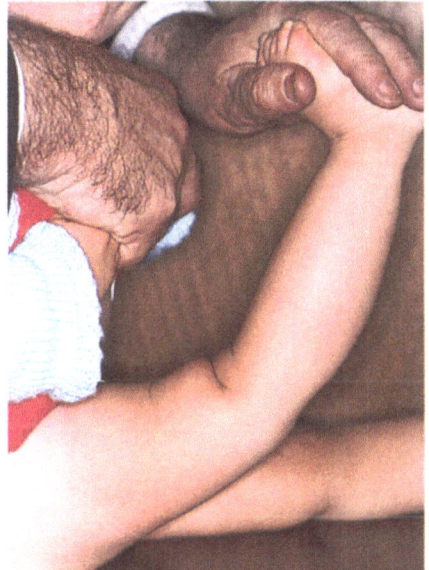

211 Age 2 years, genu recurvatum

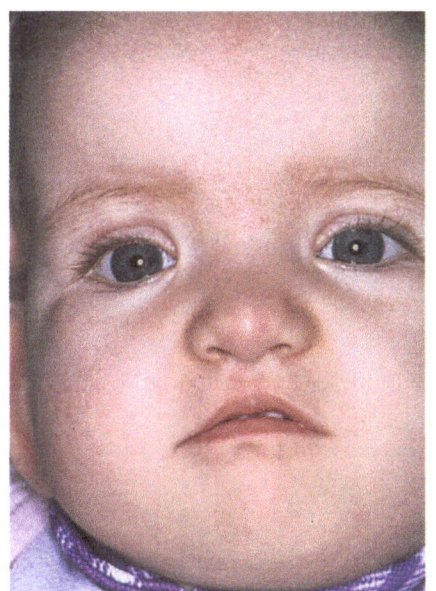

213 Age 1 year

Bilateral heterochromia

Apart from unilateral twice over, there are the great rarities of colour change spreading from the pupil in Williams' syndrome ('freckled') or in the nail-patella syndrome.

One child with nail-patella syndrome [211, 212] seemed to have a darker colour around the iris [213]; twelve years later it seems unremarkable [214], certainly not the 'dark clover leaf' one is led to expect, although she had myopic astigmatism with pigmentary retinopathy.

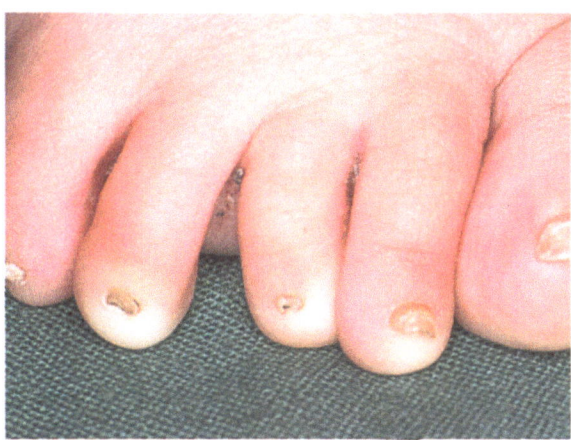

212 Age 2 years, genu recurvatum

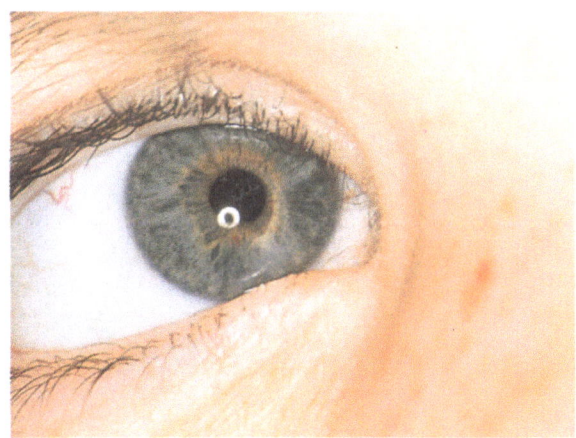

214

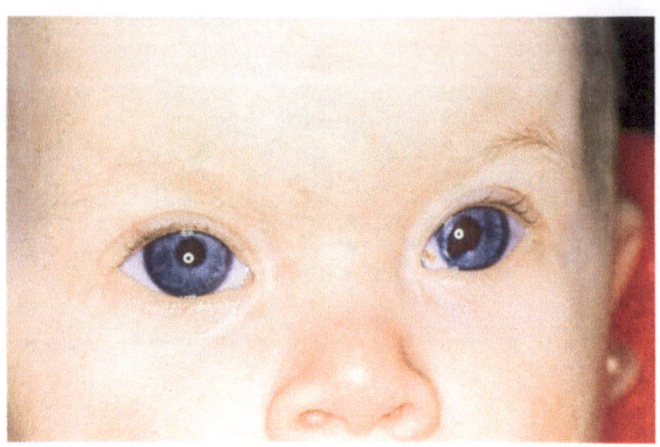

215

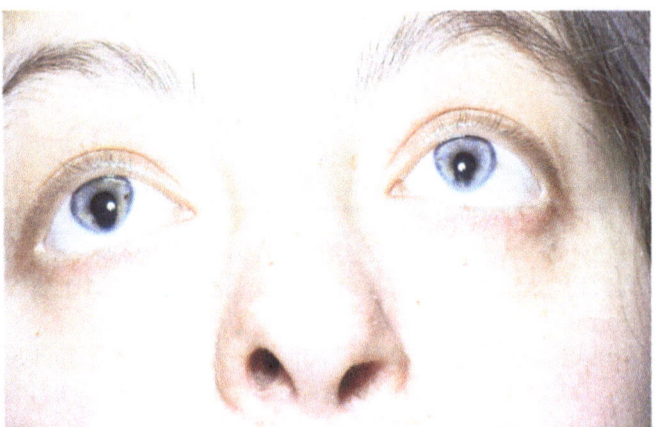

216 Antimongolian slant

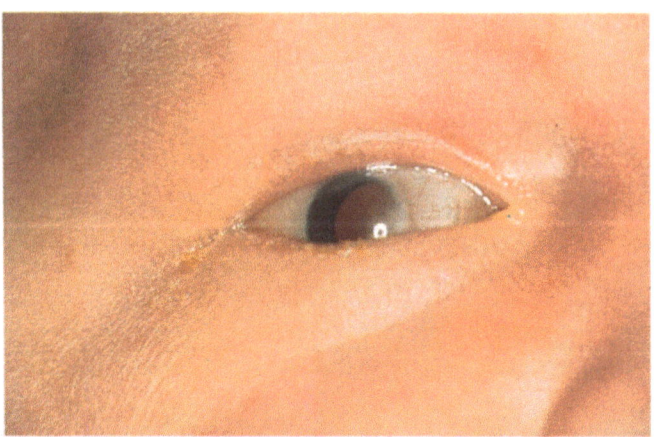

217 Coloboma with remnant of pupillary membrane on lens (and see 218)

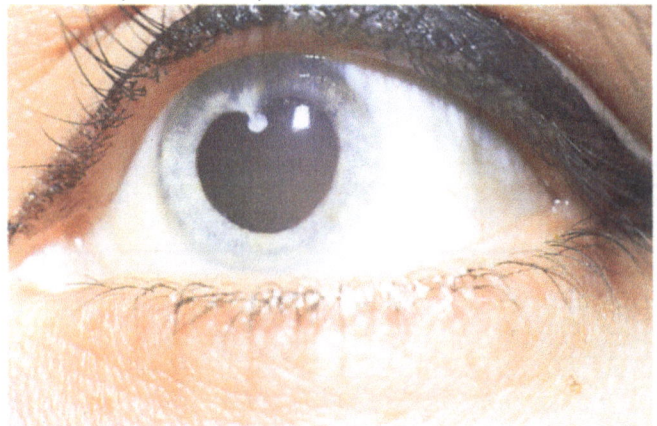

218

Lesions of the iris

The important lesion is coloboma [215] usually in the lower segment and sometimes bilateral [216]. We have seen how it could be masked [17], and how it could masquerade as a 'large pupil'; this is less likely if it is complicated [217] and/or away from its usual location.

Coloboma may be internal, affecting the fundus [see 165]; it may be more external, involving the eyelid [see 325]. It is a feature of numerous syndromes, some with chromosome abnormalities, so that karyotyping is essential.

Minor defects of the iris occur [218]; here there is a remnant of pupillary membrane attached to a subcapsular lens opacity.

Severe defects occur; *aniridia* [219] got past the vigilance of a good doctor in the nursery, presumably as 'large pupils'. Sadly, the long term outlook for vision is poor, not because of the severity of the aniridia itself but because of the associated ocular pathology. Mental handicap is common and there is a curious association with Wilms' tumour (1.5%) and finally there may be a chromosome anomaly ($11p-7$, in non-sporadic cases).

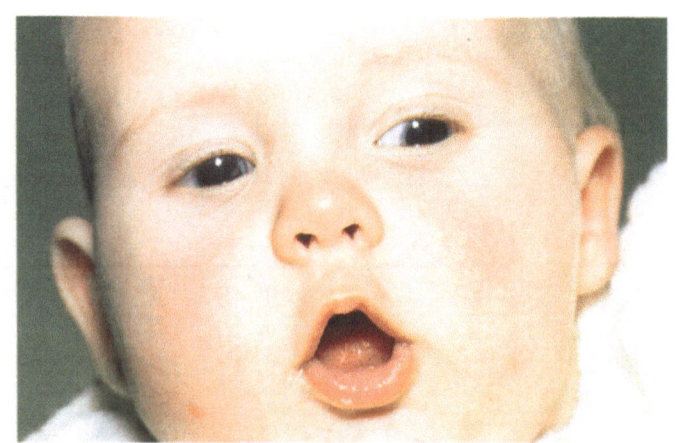

219

THE GLOBE

The common lesion is limbal dermoid [220] or dermolipoma [221]; lesions like this are still unlikely to be found in the nursery unless unusually prominent or as part of a syndrome, e.g. Goldenhar [see 351, 429]. Some are particularly well concealed [222, 223].

Blue sclerotics [224, 21] are a thin sclera that allows the venous colour to shine through, and is most commonly seen in a normal child like this. Its notoriety stems from its association with severe [225] *osteogenesis imperfecta*, but it also happens in the mild *tardive* [226] form in which case it may be expected in a parent with the appropriate history. Other inherited disorders of mesenchymal tissue, such as Marfan's syndrome [188] or *cutis laxa* show it. The clinician will of course take steps to anticipate the risk of deafness developing in affected children.

A form of conjunctival overgrowth [226A] was seen in the excessively rare *Proteus syndrome* which is characterized by indiscriminate disseminated forms of hypertrophy; this lesion was not noticed in infancy; it remains a trivial part of the overall problem.

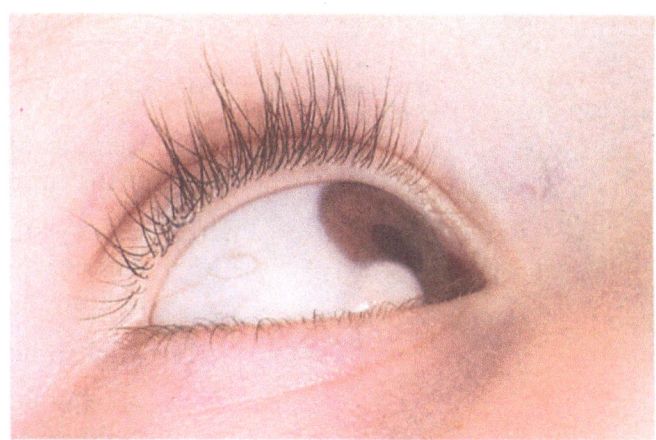

220 Age 1 year

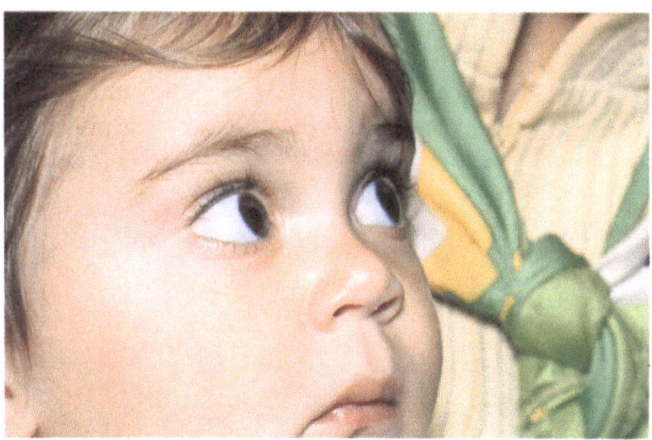

221

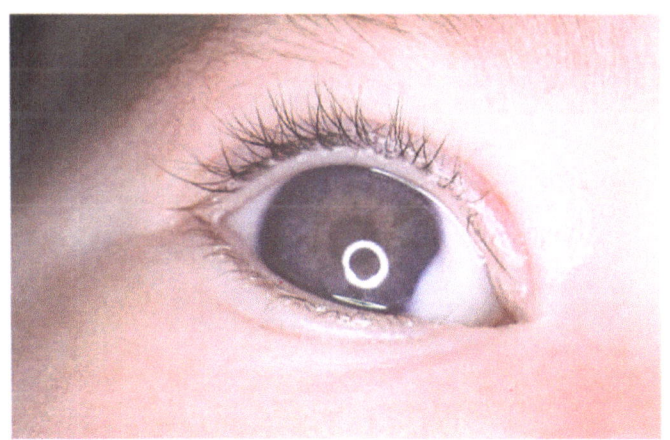

222 Age 9 months

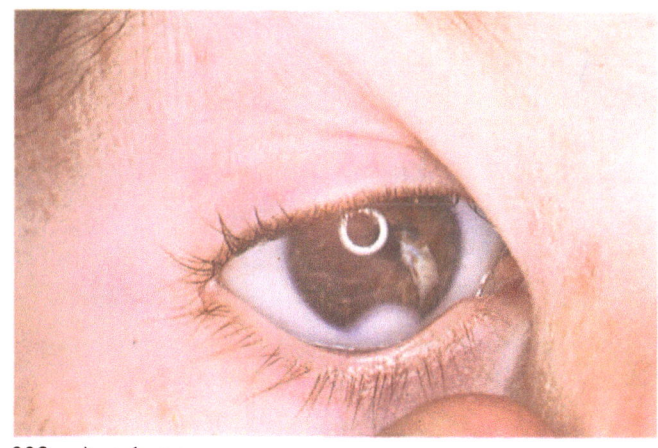

223 Age 1 year

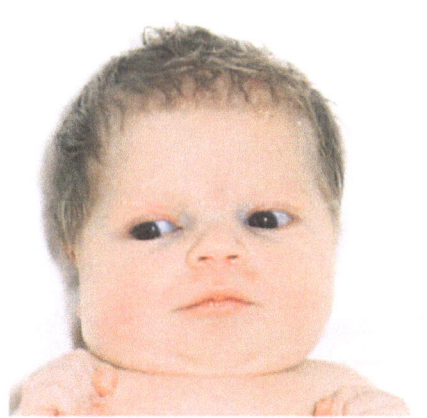

224

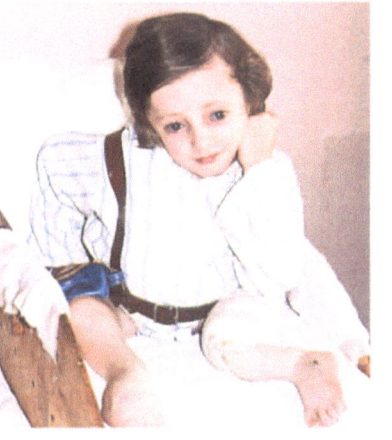

225 Age 11 years

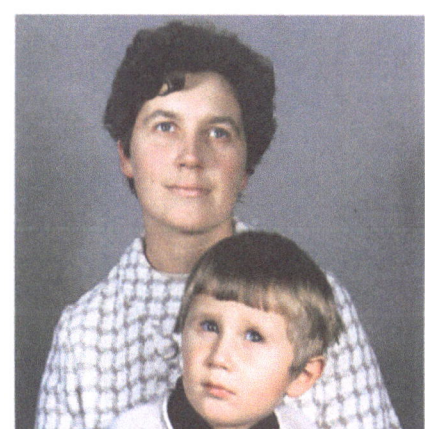

226 Tardive form

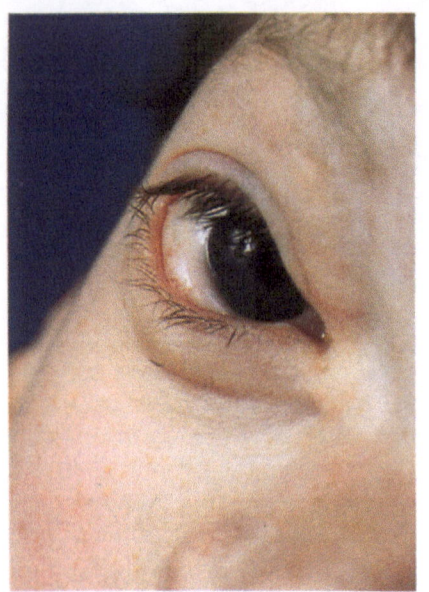

226A

THE CORNEA

Haziness is the anomaly most likely to be seen.

(1) Keratoconjunctivitis or possibly keratitis with secondary conjunctivitis, worse in the right eye, seen in a rubella baby [227].

(2) Cloudy steamy oedematous cornea of buphthalmos (ox-eye): the anterior chamber is flattened, there is epiphora. The port-wine stain indicates possible Sturge–Weber, but is masked by cosmetics [228].

(3) Mild corneal oedema, buphthalmos in Down's syndrome [229].

(4) A baby born out was admitted because of severe bilateral buphthalmos. Intraocular pressure had split the posterior surface of the cornea and aqueous humour had infiltrated forward between the layers; urgent goniotomy was required [230]. Glaucoma arising through mesodermal dysgenesis with anterior iris stroma hypoplasia and posterior corneal defects is called *Peters' anomaly*. The outlook is poor because the defective posterior cornea adheres to the lens and cataracts develop.

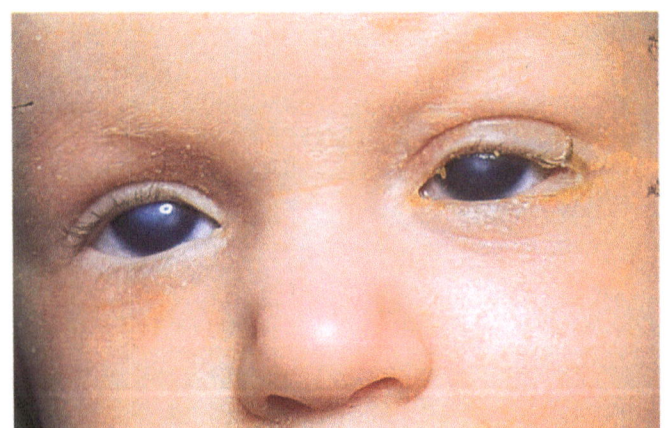

227

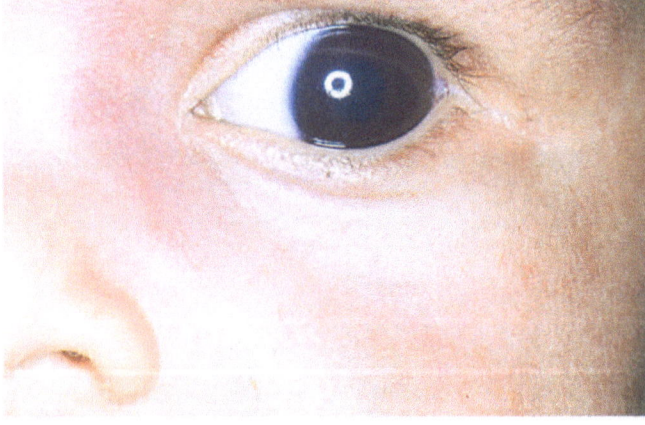

228

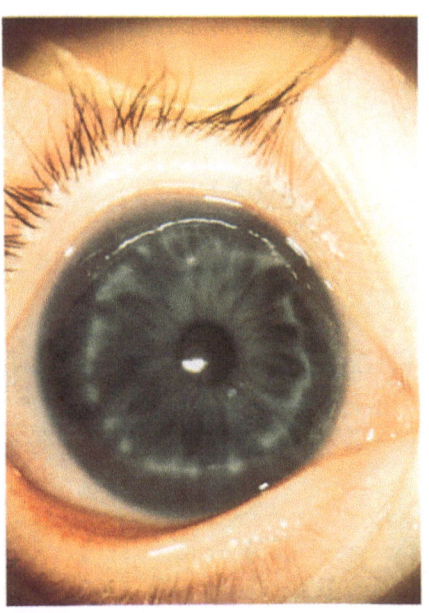

229

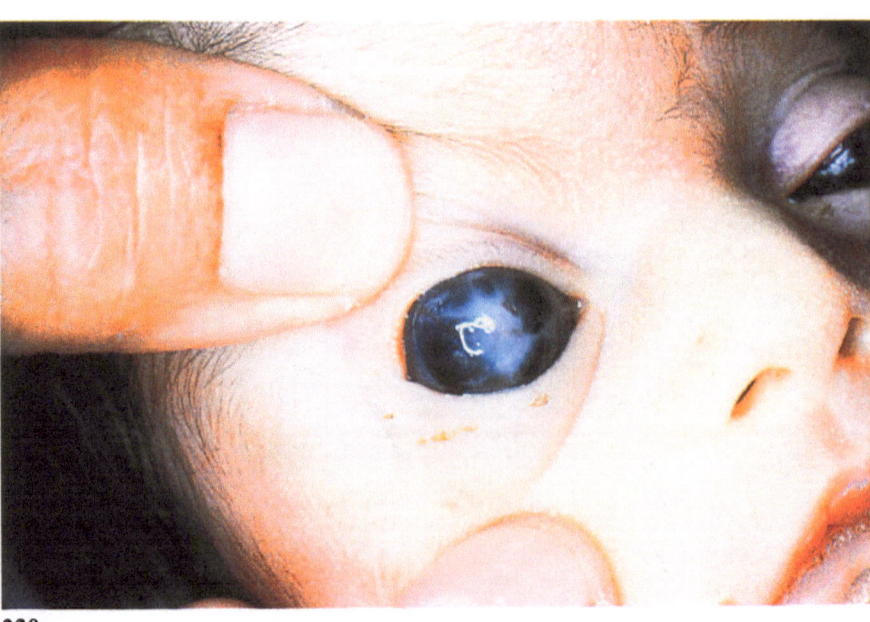

230

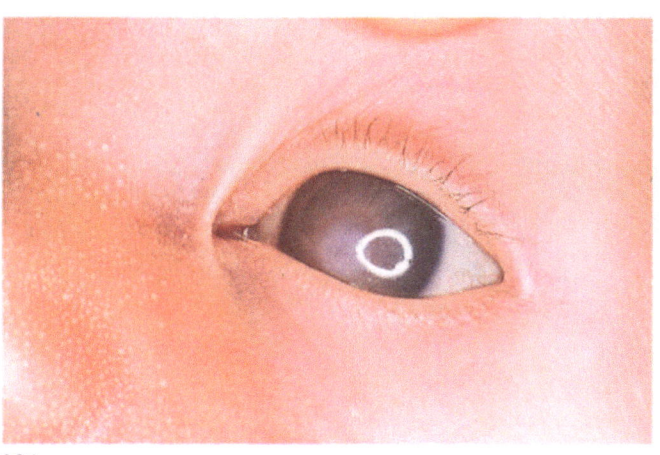

231

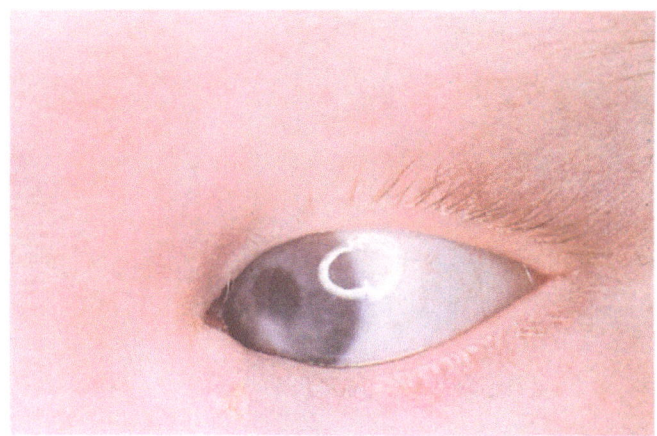

232

(5) Cloudy cornea, here the appearances suggest possible cataract with prominent iris vasculature [231]. The baby had fits but happily they stopped before long, the eye disorder cleared completely and the child is developmentally normal. In another baby [232] a white fleck was noticed by mother in the nursery but despite Down's syndrome, referral occurred only on development of a squint [233] at 8 months. The appearance is that of 'keratitis'; specialist examination showed it to be a vascular scar.

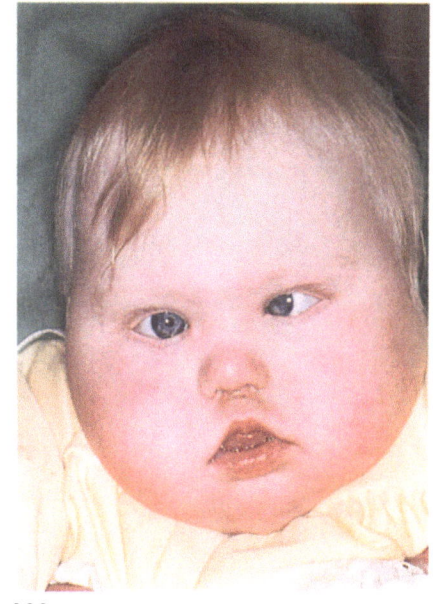

233

Congenital glaucoma may be inherited; the proof may be self-evident [234] and pre-empt the history-taking [235].

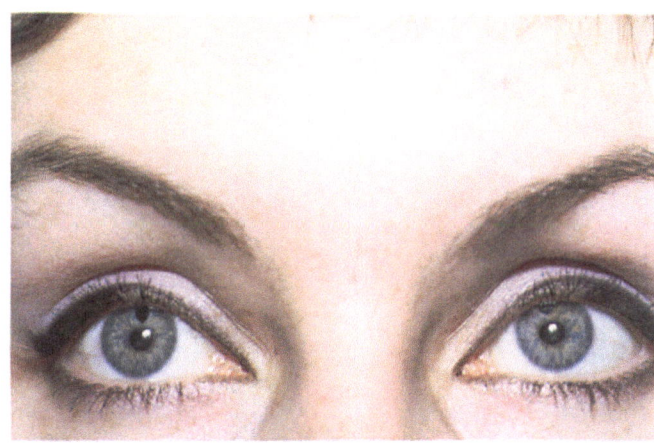

234   Bilateral iridectomy

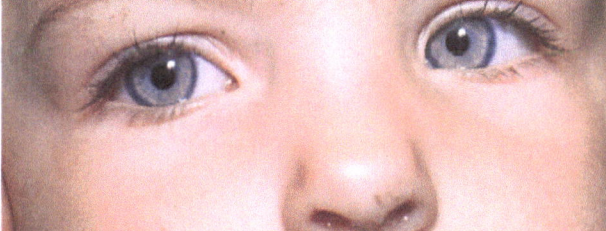

235

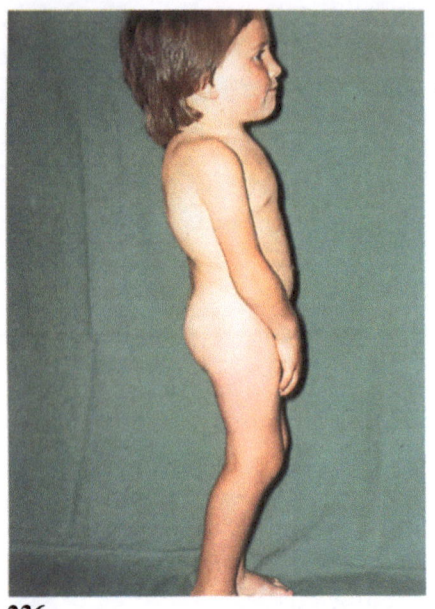

236

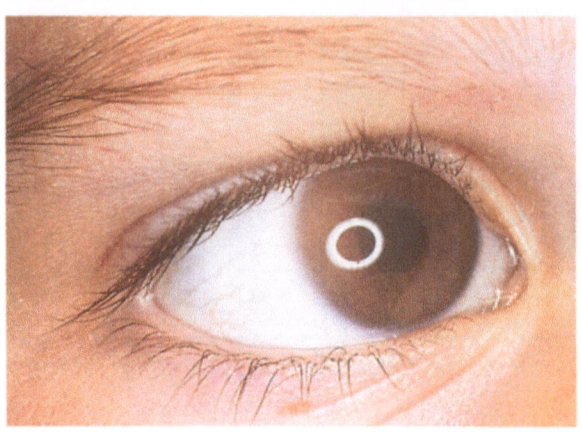

237

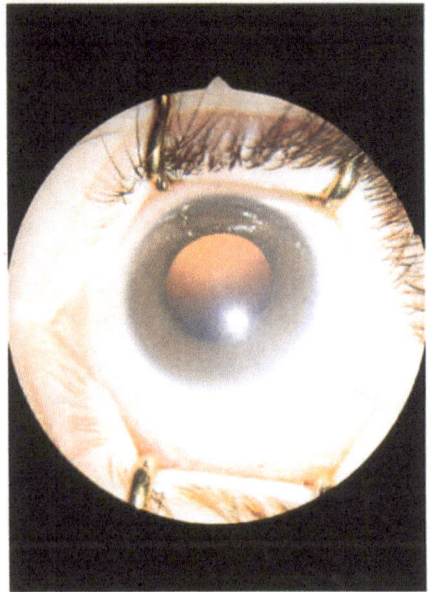

238 Age 16 months

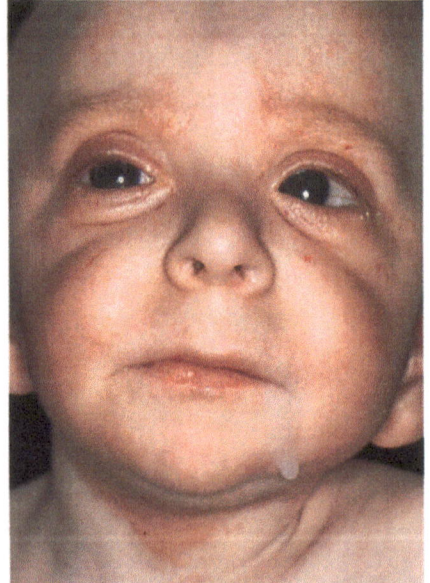

239

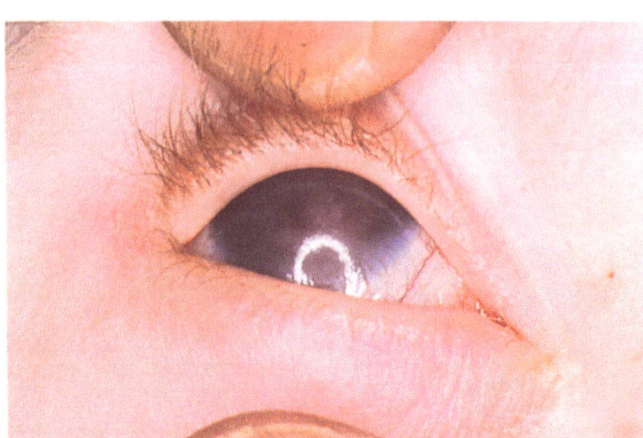

240

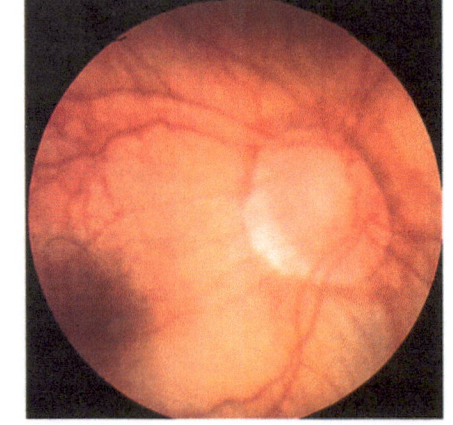

241

Hazy corneas occur in the mucopolysaccharidoses and the likelihood of congenital occurrence is remote, but the case of a Morquio child is highly relevant [236]; although her haziness was diagnosed at 5 years [237], this was the earliest possible time in its natural history, an achievement in anticipation. Cloudy corneas [238] are an important sign in Hurler's to tell it from Hunter's disease; it appears by age 3 [cf. 174]. It can be postulated that the sibling of a known Hurler will have the earliest diagnosed haziness and ultimately it may be recognized neonatally.

Anecdotal cases must abound: a boy with unexplained congenital neurological dysfunction and severe developmental delay had fairly clear corneas at 8 months [239] that became distinctly cloudy by 11 months [240]; at 3 years [241] the disk was slightly cupped with an atrophic temporal crescent, the fundus lightly pigmented. CT scan shows moderate ventricular dilatation. Our battery of diagnostic investigations has drawn a blank.

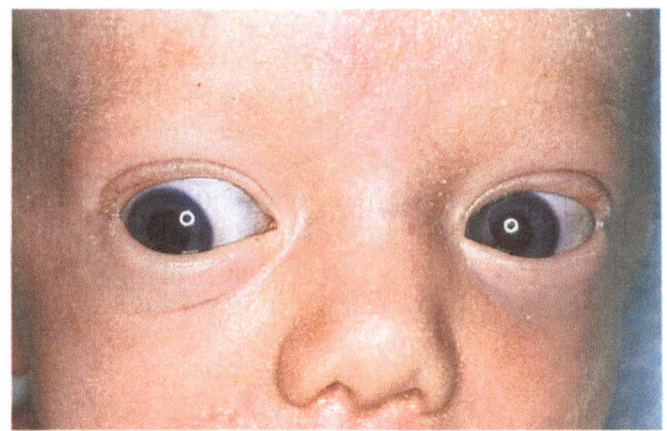

242

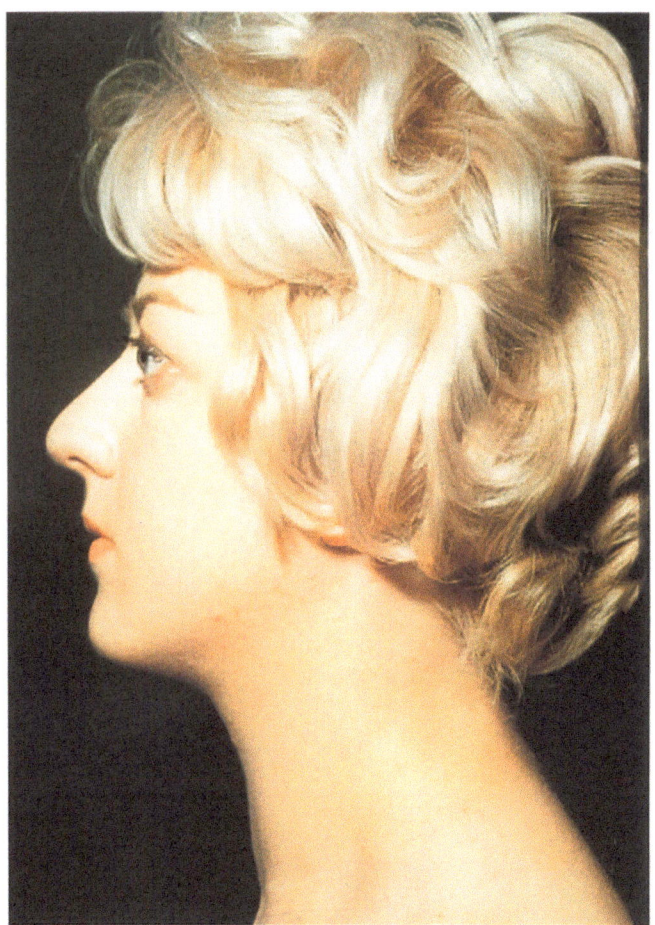

243

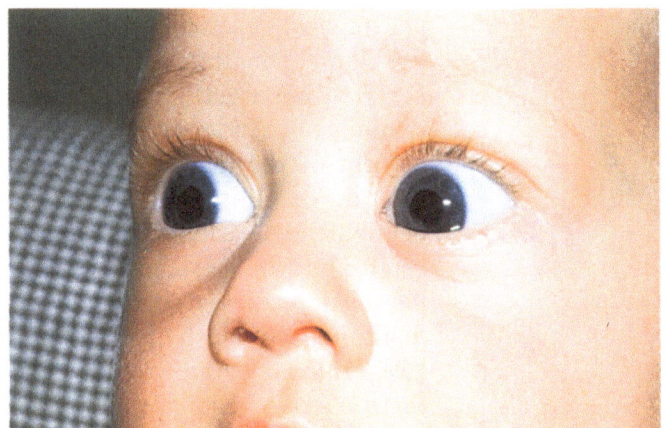

244

PROMINENT EYES

Exophthalmos [242] may identify the hyperthyroid baby, in this instance the mother was herself exophthalmic [243], having had an operation for Graves's disease. It is mothers like this with an elevated serum level of LATS and related antibodies who have babies at risk. The baby's exophthalmos persisted for many months [244]; during this time she showed a transient 'setting sun sign'.

A girl with prominent eyes at birth still shows it at 12 years [245]; a smooth non-toxic goitre developed in recent months and she is prepubertal.

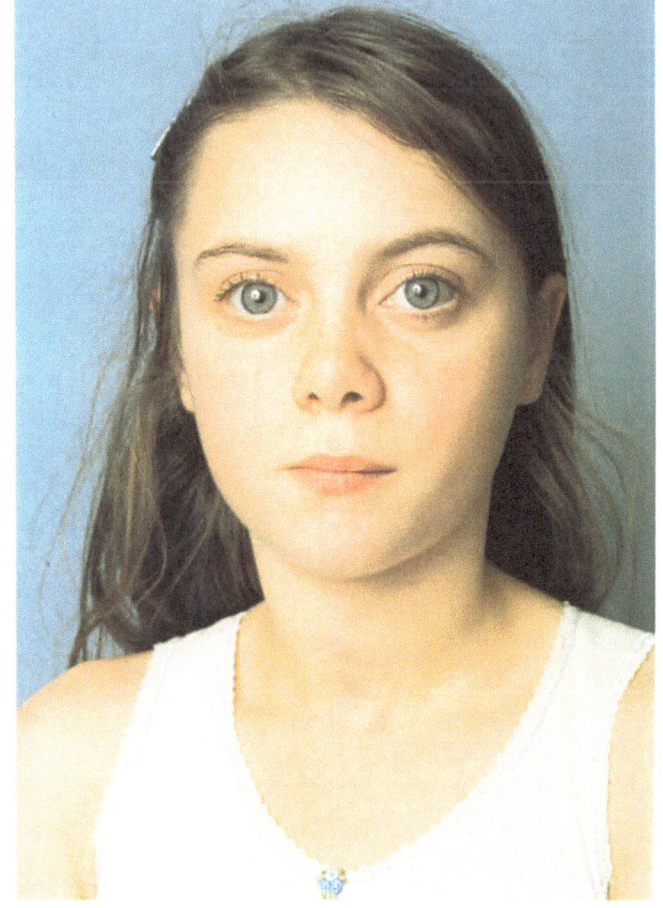

245

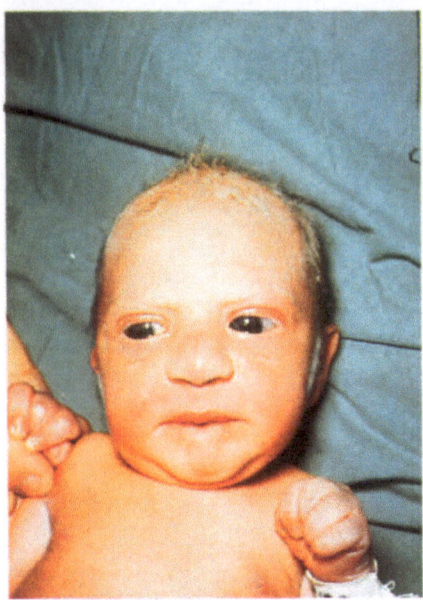

246 Note fisting

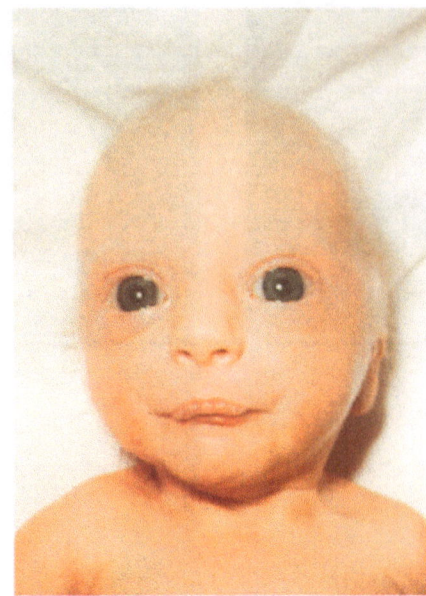

247

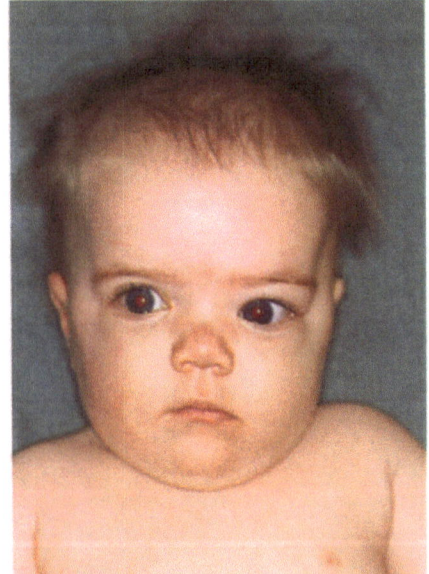

248

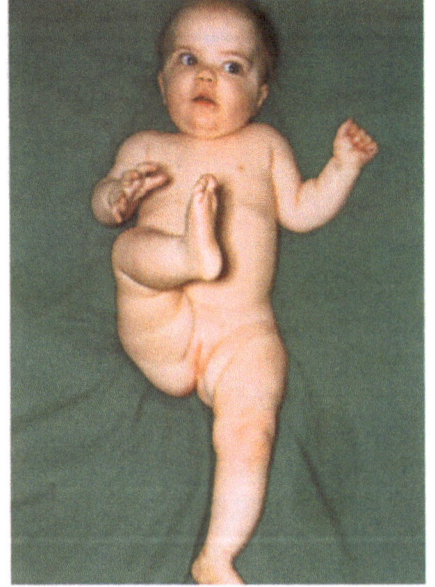

249

A microcephalic baby had prominent eyes [246] and a similar sibling was spastic in addition [247]. Subsequently they were both found to have *alaninuria*.

A baby born with one displaced prominent eye [248] was not referred until age 8 months. There was obvious hemiparesis [249] and some café-au-lait [250] spots; *von Recklinghausen's neuroectodermal dysplasia* was diagnosed, there were typical X-ray changes in limb bones and a plexiform neuroma was excised. The eye was too large for the normal orbit [251], apparently megalophthalmos or pseudobuphthalmos as a form of the local gigantism so typical of this disorder. The hemiparesis was from middle cerebral artery stenosis [252], happily it recovered completely. In due course brownish *Lisch nodules* [see 210], appeared in both eyes; there is a remote risk of malignant melanoma developing.

Prominent eyes are also a feature of Crouzon's disease [see 303–318] and related disorders with shallow orbits.

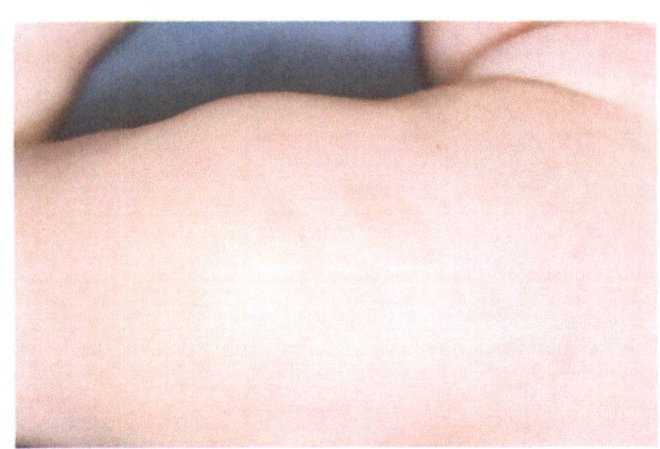

250 Café-au-lait spots

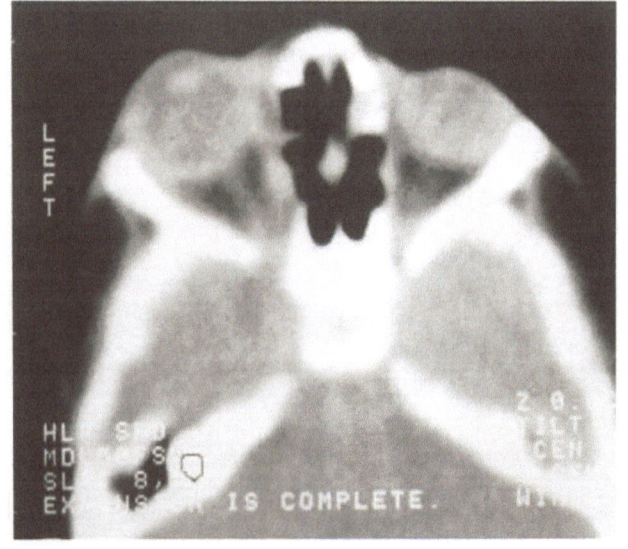

251

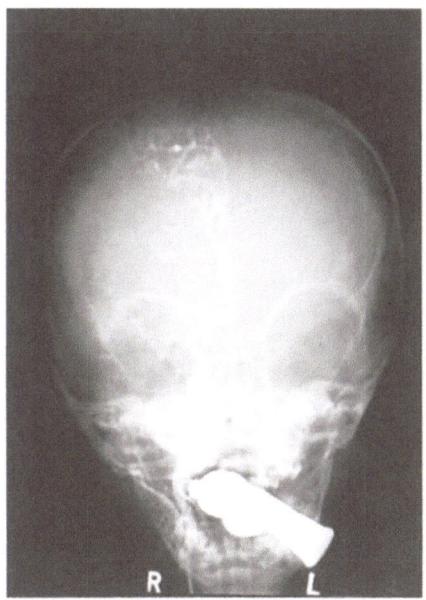

252 Avascular territory

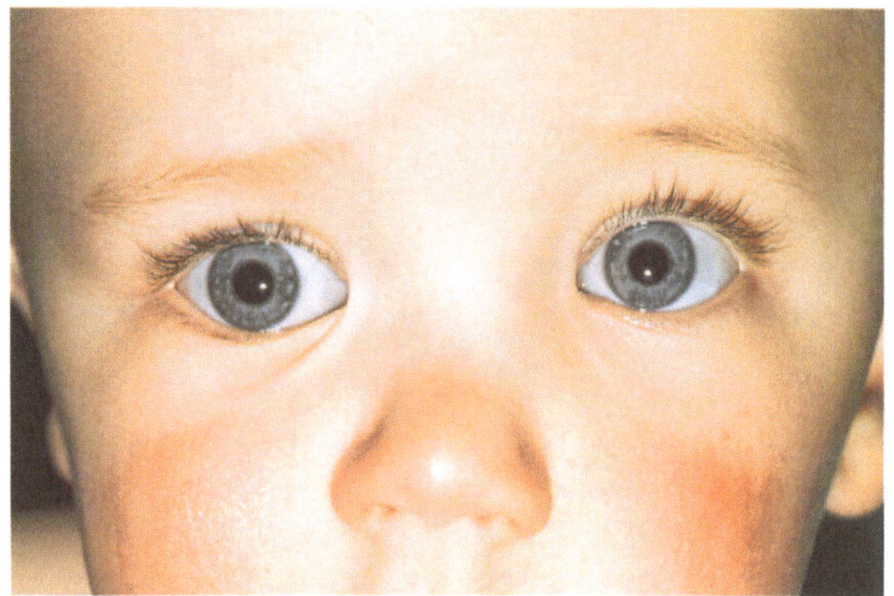

253 Age 10 months

Two cases of displaced eye may be included here, they were at least prominent in the parents' minds. They were both noticed at birth, the first was seen at 10 months [253], the surgeon found there was premature fusion of the coronal suture. Six months later there was a distinct improvement [254] that handsomely vindicated his conservative policy. The second baby was dealt with at primary care level and is happy [255] in his minimal asymmetry.

Premature fusion of one [256] or both coronal sutures is the commonest finding in true plagiocephaly; nowadays the CT scan [257] is a source of further information.

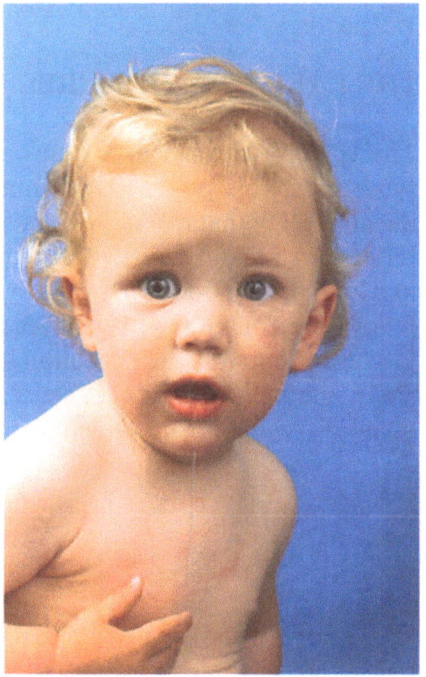
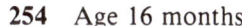

254 Age 16 months

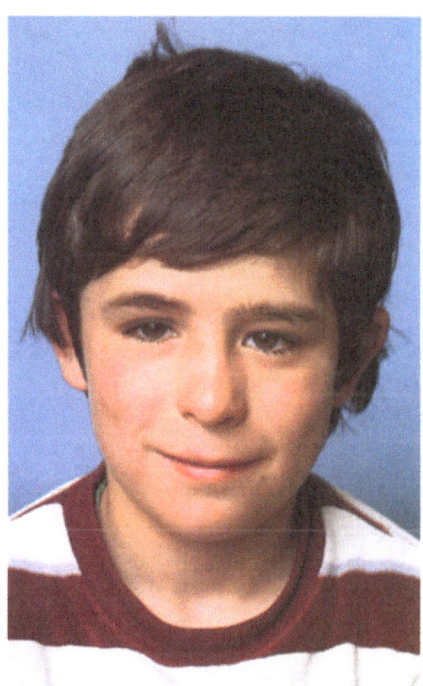

255

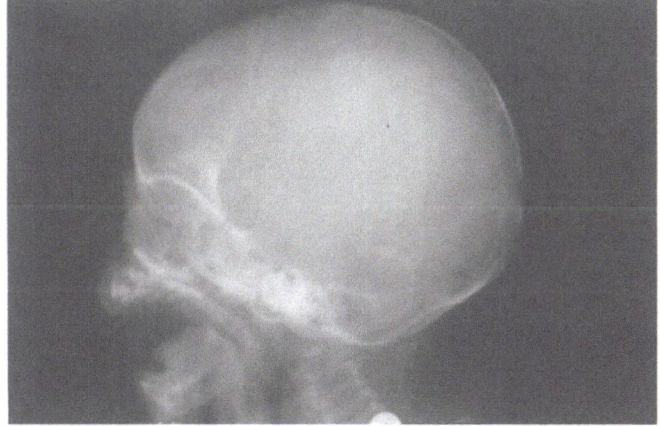

256 Short straight right coronal suture with sclerotic margin

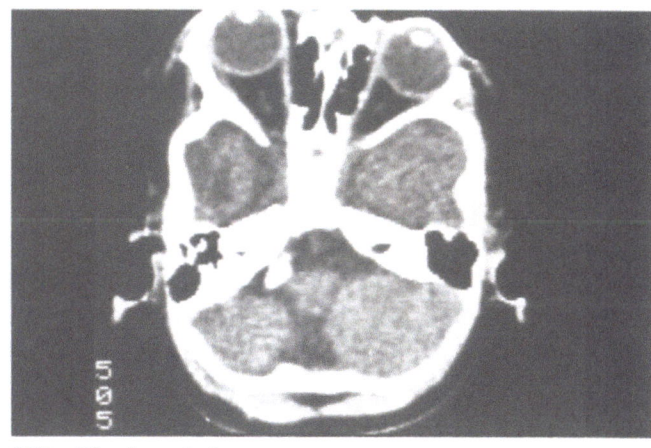

257 Plagiocephaly

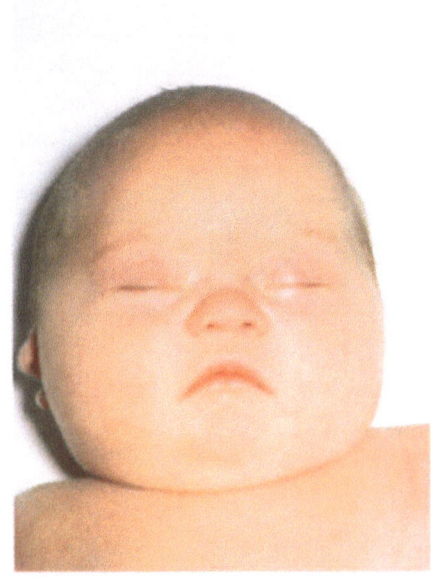

258 Note carp mouth

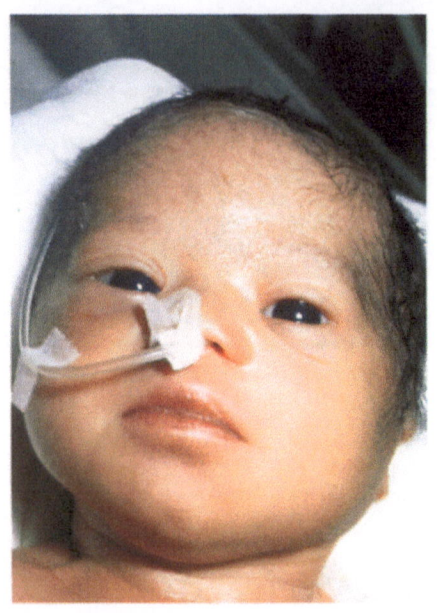

259 Same baby as in **53**.
Admixture West Indies/Irish

THE PALPEBRAL FISSURES

The celebrated anomaly is upward mongolian slant [258] in Down's syndrome. This goes with prominent epicanthic fold and broad root of the nose [259] that often give a false appearance of squint, but the corneal reflections are our guide. Before long, in fact, squint [260] does develop in a high proportion of Down's syndrome children. A prominent slant in a normal neonate may be misleading initially.

The commonest cause of mongolian slant is of course being a Mongol [261], the next commonest cause is being a half-caste [262]. Note their facial difference from Down's syndrome.

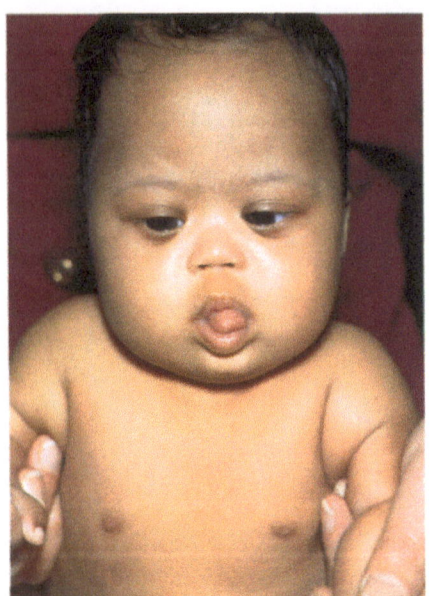

260 Same baby, 3 months

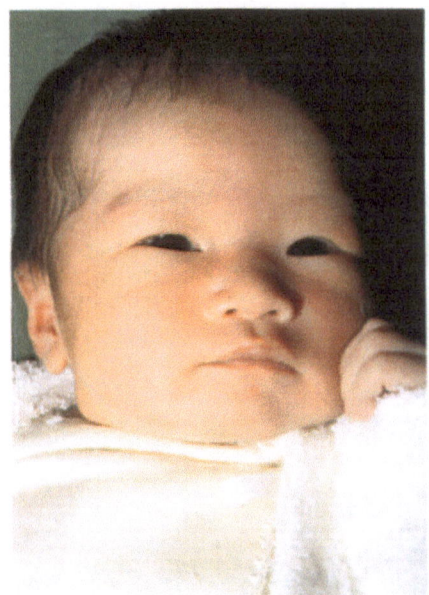

261 Chinese

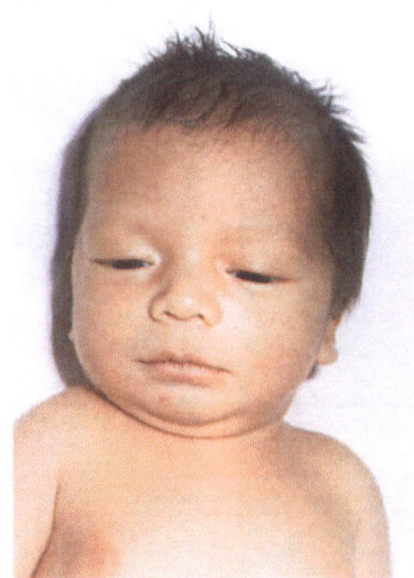

262 Anglo-Burmese

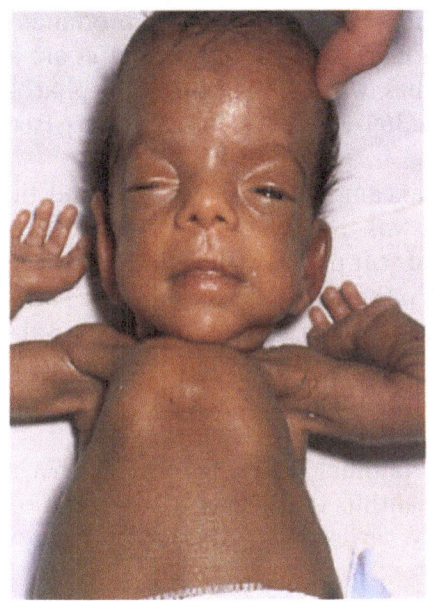

263 A pre-term baby

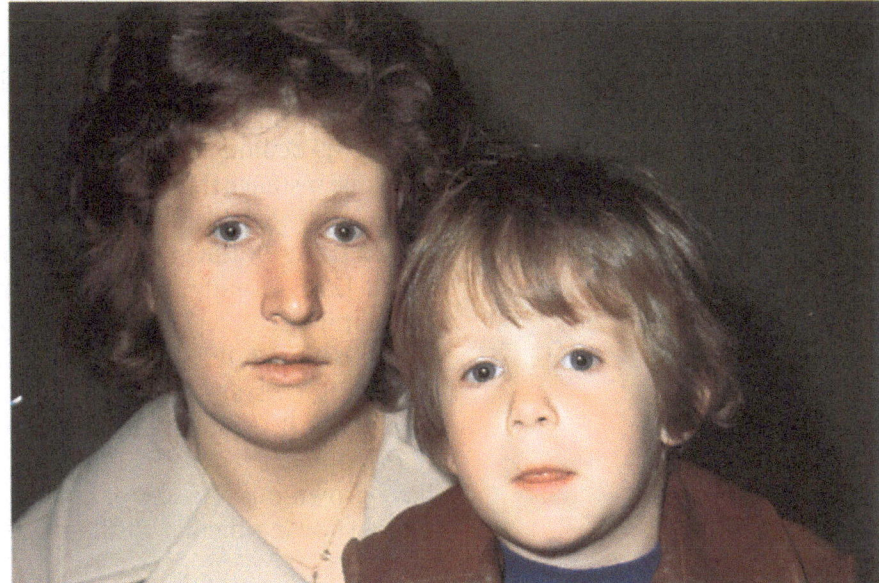

264

Antimongolian downward slant features in many syndromes, especially with facial dysostosis, but it is commonest in normal children [263] although sometimes with divergent squint like this baby's. It may also be familial [264]. Antimongolian slant in one case [265] is overshadowed by the deep nasal notching typical of Warfarin embryopathy; there are hypoplastic nails [266, 267] and short fingers.

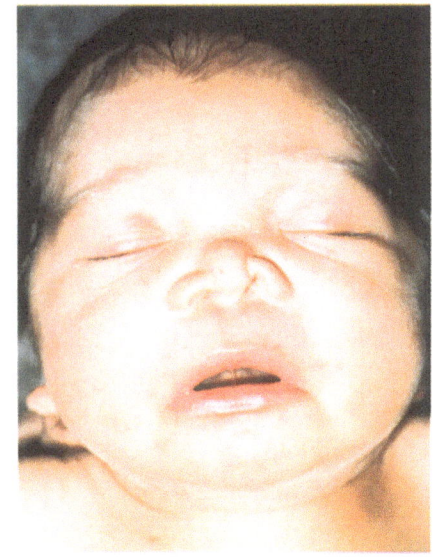

265 Notched nostrils led to recognition of Warfarin embryopathy (1970)

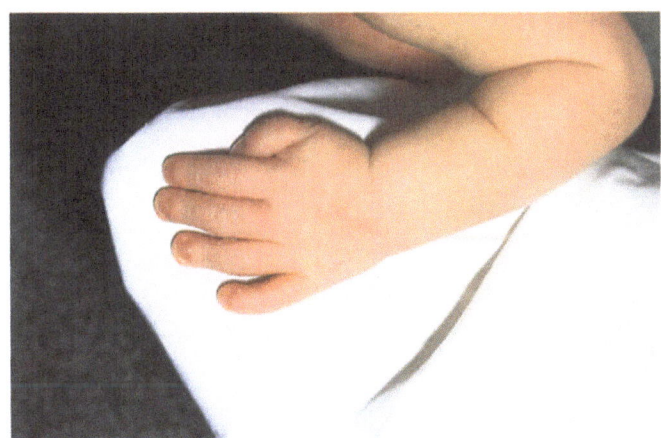

266

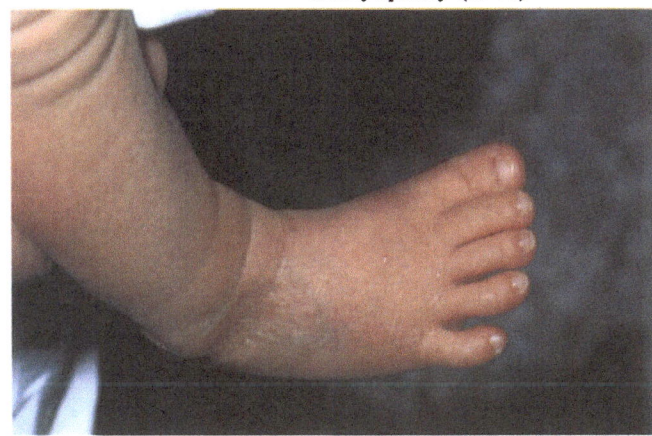

267

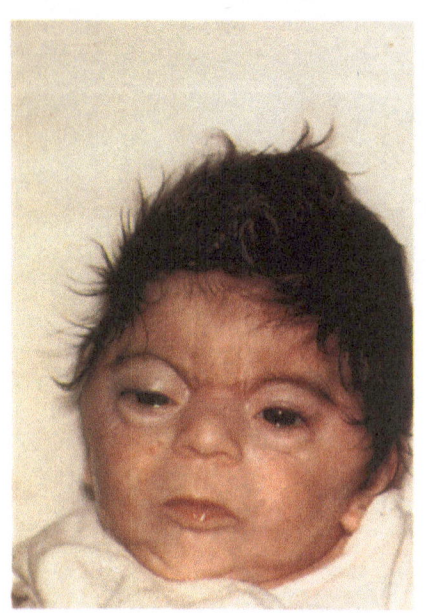

Short palpebral fissures with synophrys [268] are relatively prominent in the de Lange/phenytoin/fetal alcohol syndromes. Short fissures are a mild stigma of several other syndromes with telecanthus – blepharophimosis [91, 92], midline cleft face [see 365–367, 389], Waardenburg [see 331–334], oculodentodigital [335].

In one instance this was the stigma that came in last, since the diagnostic drive was centripetal. First noticed was polysyndactyly [269], then irregularities of the alveolar margin and soft palate with inclusions in the uvula [270], finally partial cleft mid upper lip, telecanthus and short palpebral fissures [271]. All together, in proper order, this is the *oral-facial-d*igital (OFD type I), typically affecting a girl. Expert genetic advice is necessary, especially as hallux reduplication is more typical of OFD type II (Mohr).

Prominent epicanthic folds may be familial [272]; here the mother's have grown out and she has mild telecanthus that leaves a good deal of sclera showing medial to the iris (see Waardenburg, 333).

268

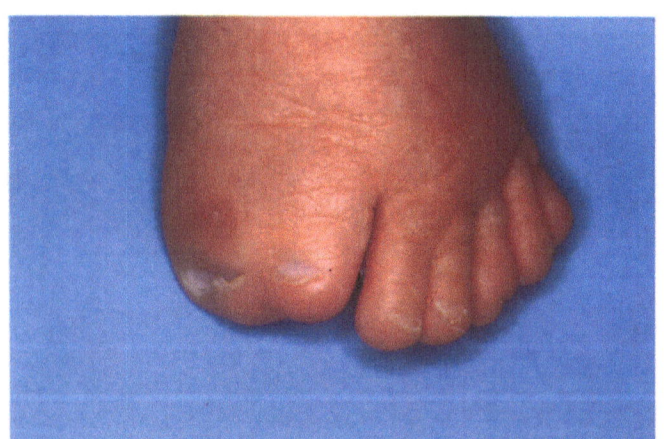

269   Hallux reduplication

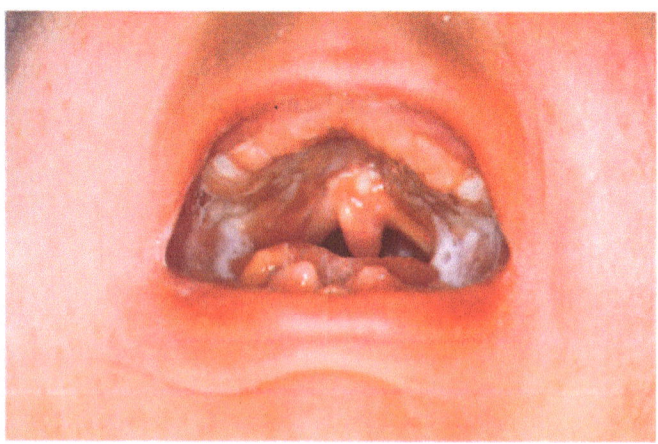

270

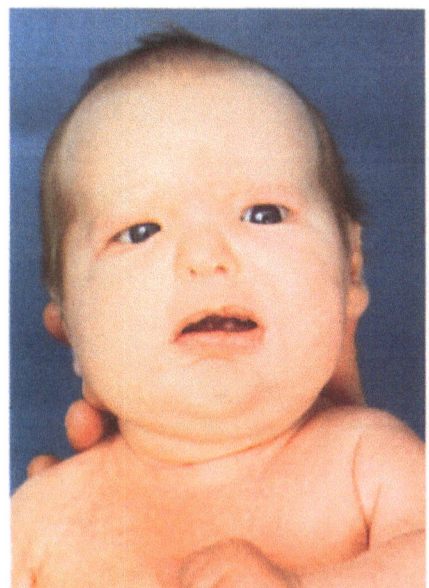

271   *cf.* Smith, D. 3rd edition, 1982, p.191 (Saunders)

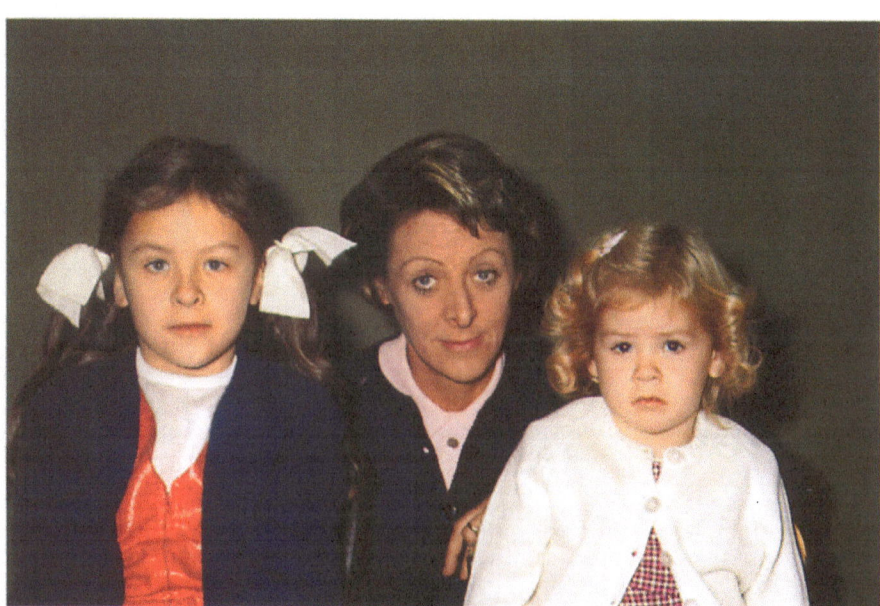

272

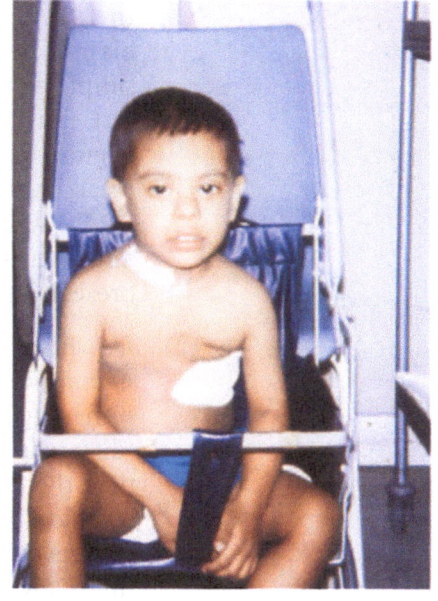

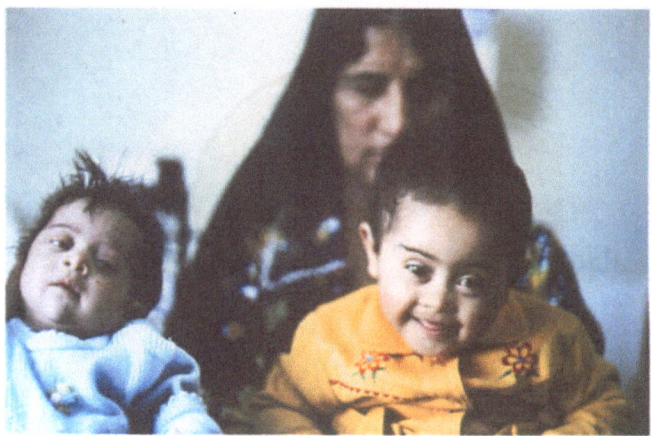

273 Down's syndrome in a twin, the telecanthus and hypotelorism is not usually part of Down's and in this case was inherited from the father

274 Siblings 13th, 14th

Down's syndrome plus. Three classical conundrums

There are three possible areas of clinical confusion; the passage of time has rendered them less hazardous due to a combination of familiarity and technology:

(1) *Down's syndrome in the non-caucasian* was thought to be possibly rare or subtle until the secondment of non-consultant paediatricians in training to Africa in the 1950s proved there was no great problem [273] of supply or diagnosis. The Muslim world was little different [274]; in this instance recognition was sadly facilitated through an affected sibling. At home, mutual sociability produced the half-caste case [275], West Indies and Westmeath in this instance. The big one, of course, is Down's in an Oriental, and there is now a local supply from our Boat People [276]. If tradition is honoured by attending to the eye signs the nuances are there, the double line of the upper lid [277] as well as the depressed rather than flat nasal bridge [278].

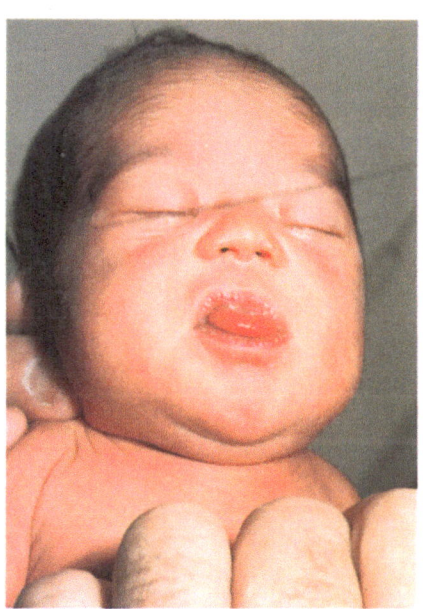

275

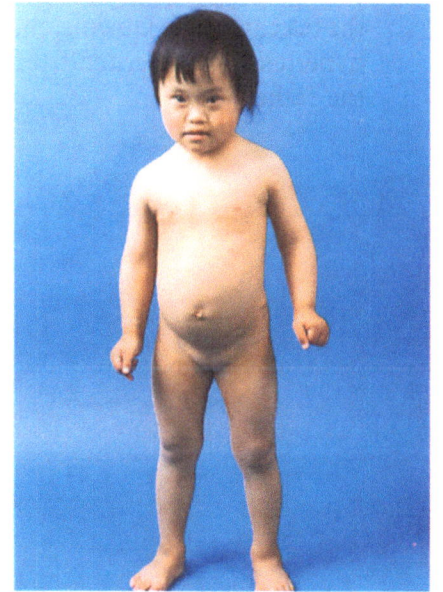

276 Vietnamese Down's . . .

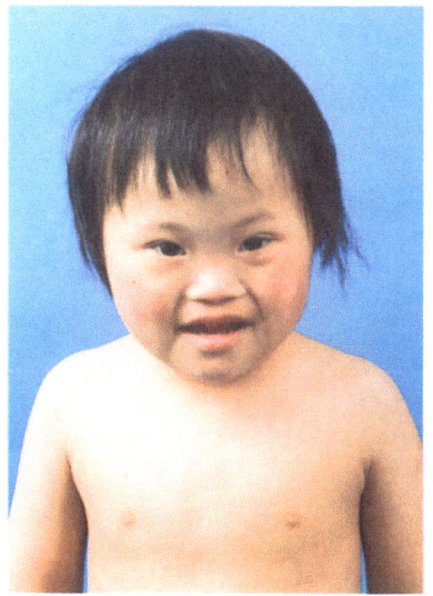

277 Has depressed nasal bridge . . .

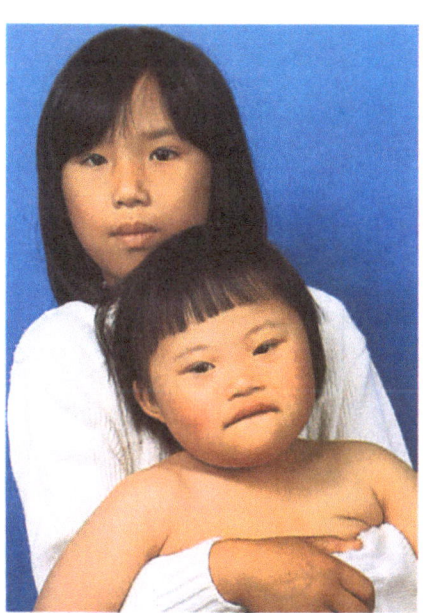

278 Unlike normal sibling

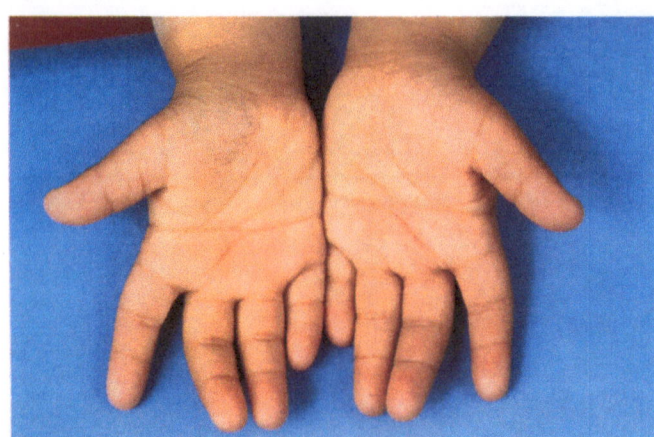

279

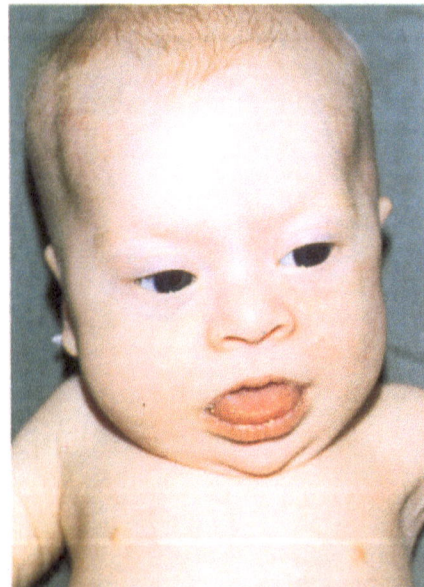

280 Age 7 weeks

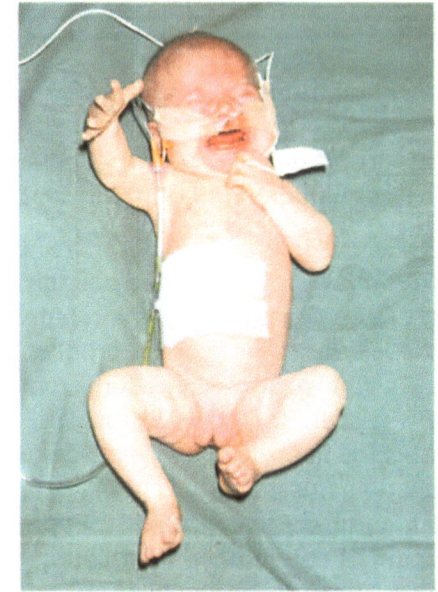

281 Age 19 days

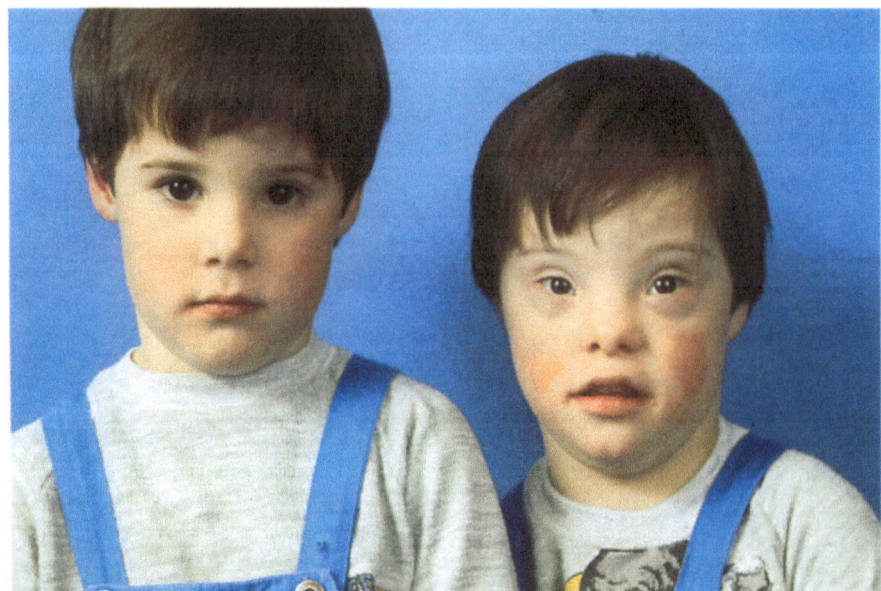

282 Age five years

In fact a better index is the pinna, always small and of simple configuration; for the rest it is the other familiar stigmas of hypotonia, simian creases and short little fingers [**279**], with broad toe cleft and intestinal anomaly in the present instance.

(2) *Down's syndrome with hypothyroidism* once had some vogue as an unrealistic 'differential diagnosis' poser, then there was a brief period of one-off curiosity-type case reports until it was realised that Down's is indeed linked with thyroid disorders; 1% are either hypothyroid (athyreosis) or hyperthyroid or else have simple goitre. Early clinical diagnosis can be very challenging [**280**] but even if we remarked this rather floppy tongue to the more usual busy darting one [**see 275**], the diagnosis was long established thanks to universal neonatal screening. In the neonatal period the Down's duodenal atresia was operated [**281**]; maybe there were hypothyroid clues in the ready periorbital oedema and largish tongue.

(3) *Down's syndrome with tele-canthus and hypertelorism:* the telecanthus is Down's, the hypertelorism inherited from the father [**282**].

THE EYELIDS

Epiphora due to entropion [283, 284] was noticed in the nursery by the mother; at 8 months in the health centre she had to draw it to the doctor's attention following a routine examination. The ophthalmologist saw that the cornea had no abrasions from the soft lashes so he waited, but after 2 months needed to cauterize the lower lid [285] to evert the lashes.

Epiphora from birth in a girl of 5 [286] was associated with paucity of lower lid lashes and there was absence of the nasolacrimal punctum [287]. This was Treacher Collins syndrome in a very mild form; she has slight mandibulofacial hypoplasia.

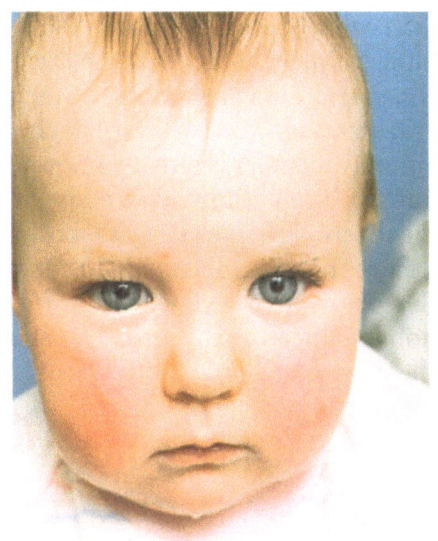

283

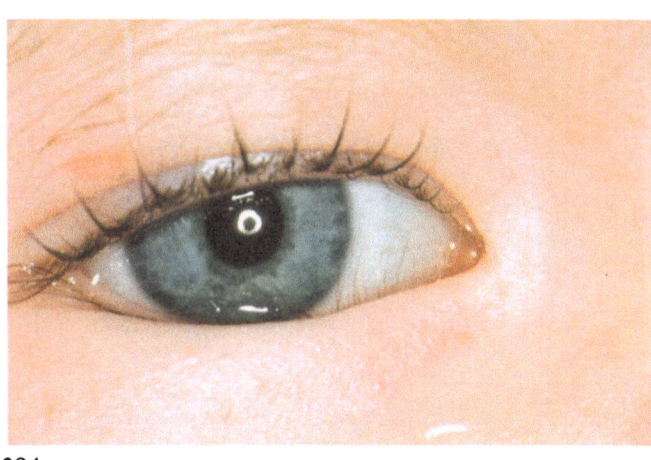

284

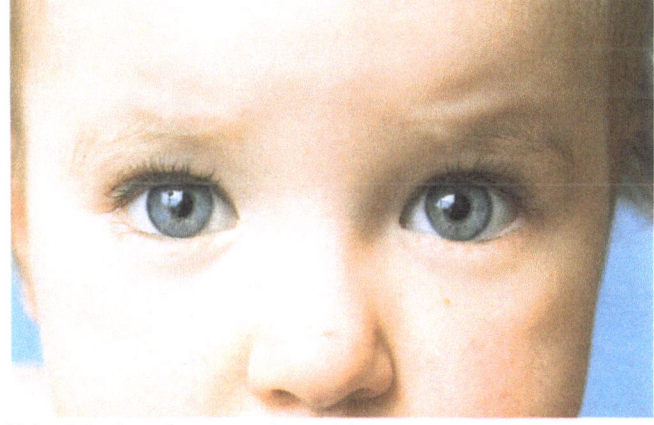

285 Marks of cautery just visible

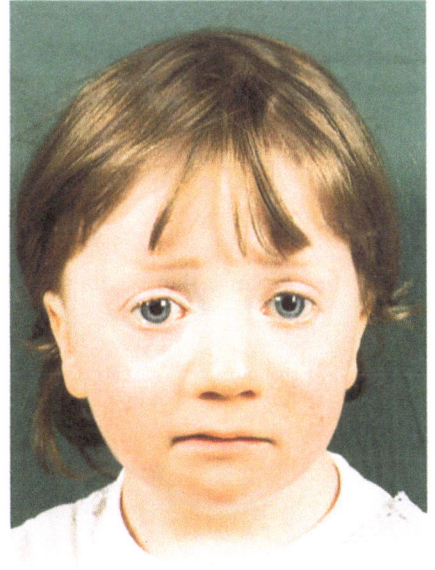

286

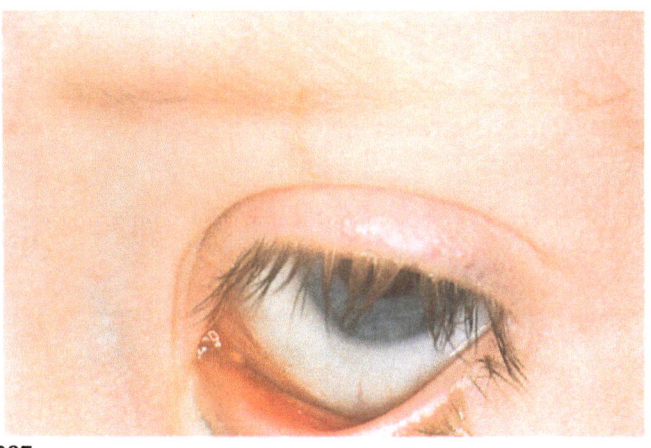

287

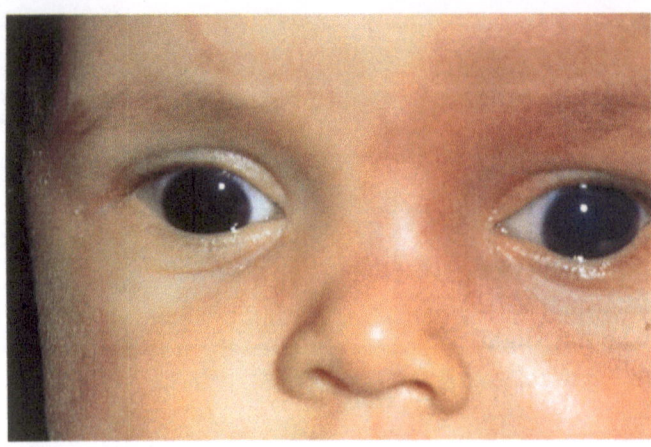

288

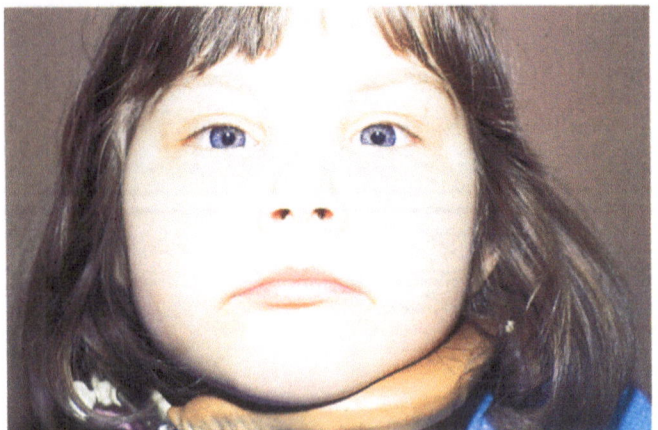

289 Slight crusting on lids

In a neonate, epiphora [288] drew attention to buphthalmos; there is corneal cloudiness. The portwine stain indicates possible Sturge–Weber disease.

Absence of tears will very likely go unnoticed unless a family member is already known [289], as in this case due to *Riley–Day dysautonomia*. The new baby's diagnosis was nevertheless postneonatal [290, 291] because no-risk advice was mistakenly given, in spite of the descriptive byline *congenital familial* dysautonomia indicating the recessive inheritance. Dryness of the cornea and conjunctiva causes photophobia; they may not shed tears.

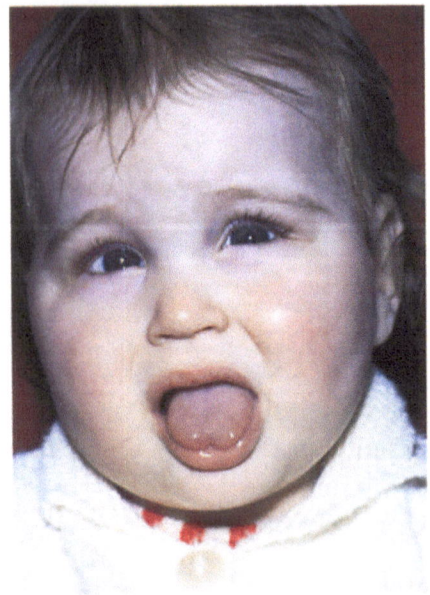

290 Note eyes screwed up . . .

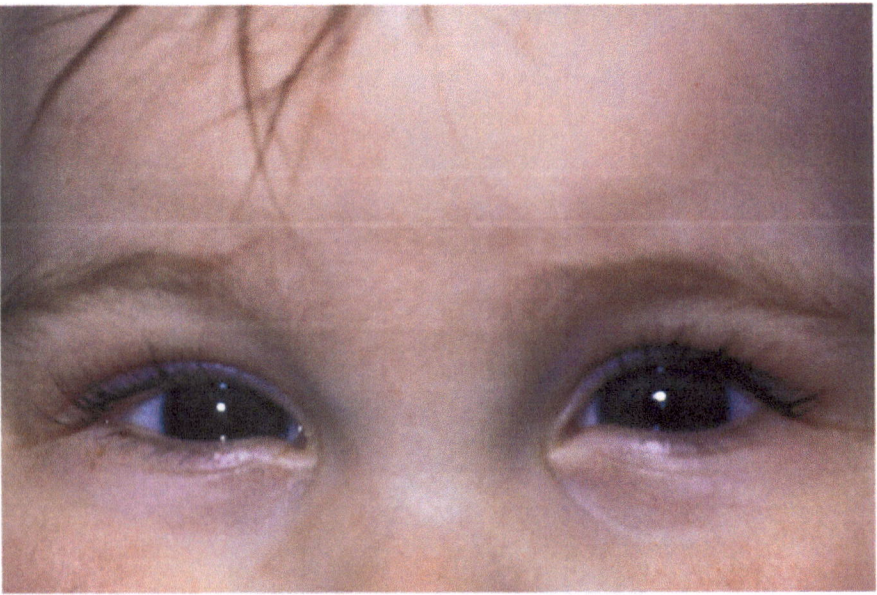

291 Lashes may injure cornea because there is pain insensitivity

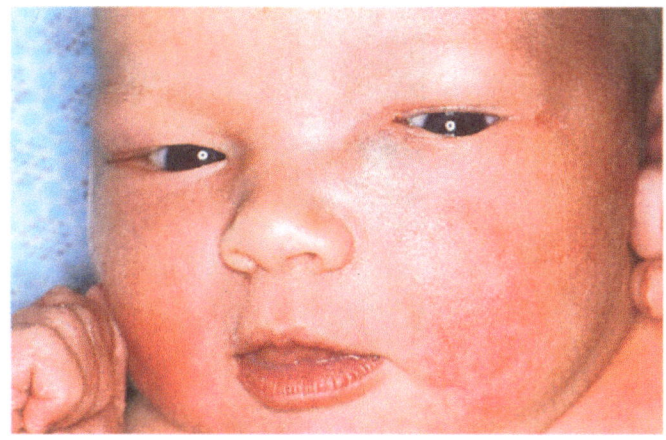

292

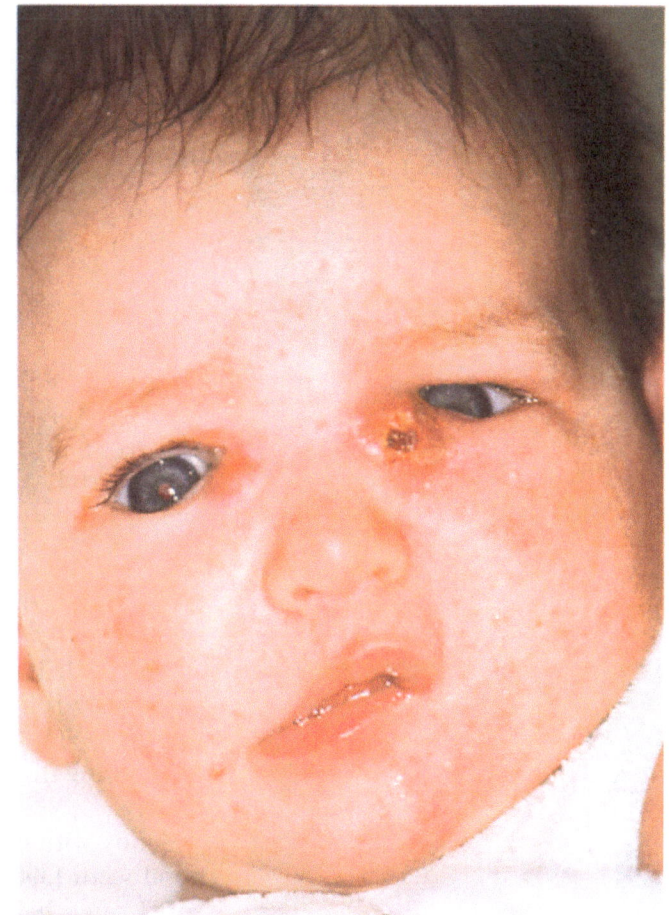

293

Medial swelling over the nasolacrimal duct is most likely mucocele [292]; there is risk of infection and abscess may develop [293] unless something is done.

Lateral swelling in this position [294] is usually external angular dermoid, surgical removal is done after the first birthday, for cosmetic reasons.

Absence of eyelashes and eyebrows [295] with skin that quickly goes dry [296] points to congenital ectodermal dysplasia, but it usually takes an affected

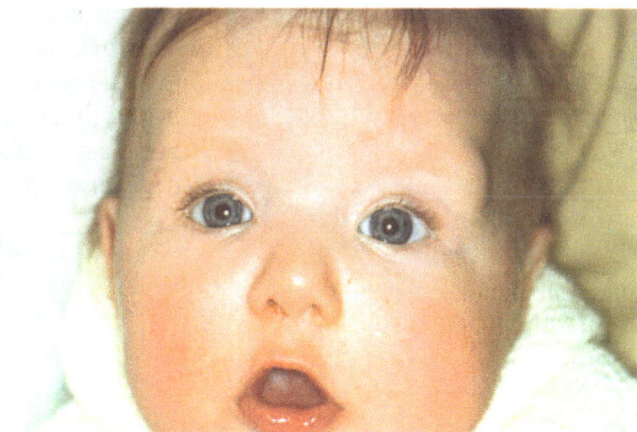

294   Typical location

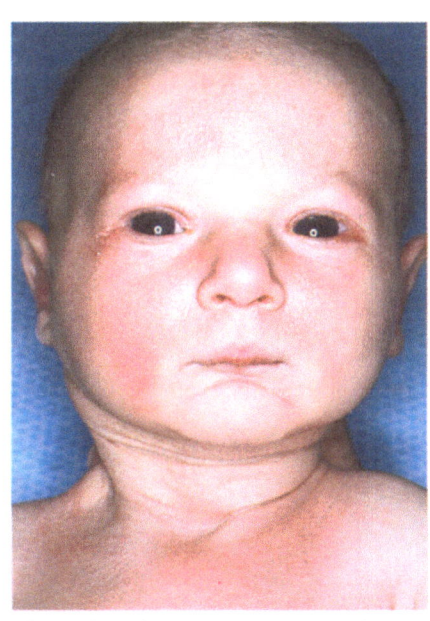

295   First day, note 'dummy' look

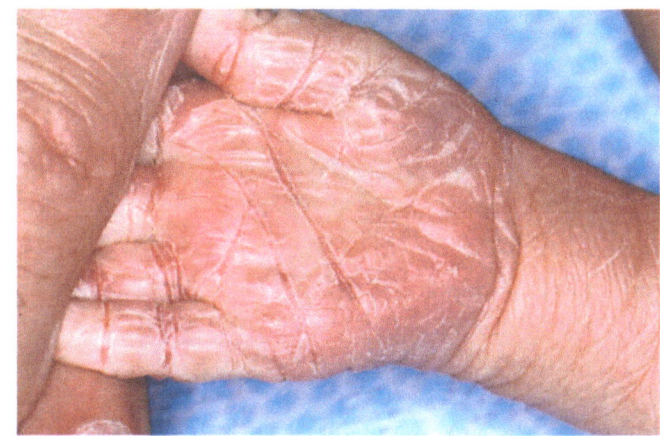

296   Second day

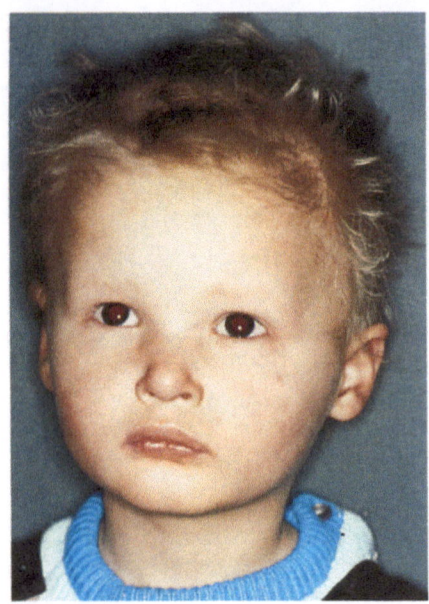

297 Age 20 months, hair fairly well grown

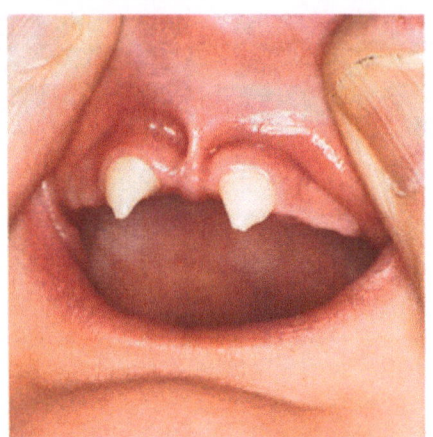

298 Teeth are few, conical. Dental referral necessary

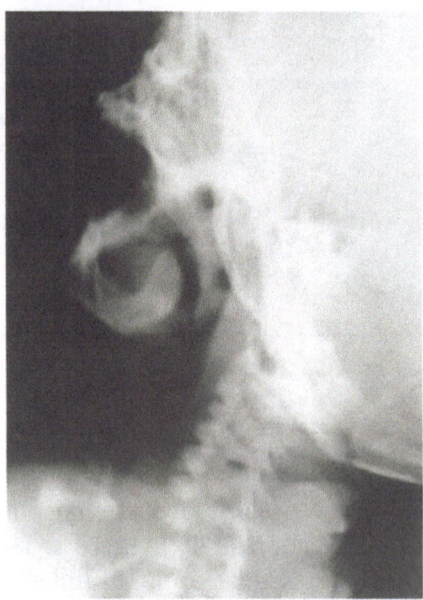

299

sibling [297, 298] to achieve the clinical diagnosis in the nursery, then this is easily corroborated by the absence of dental sacs [299] in the X-ray of mandible. The sibling was known to be *hydrotic* so there was the relief of knowing that the baby had therefore not got the dangerous *anhydrotic* variety.

A boy with hypohydrotic ectodermal dysplasia has total alopecia with good teeth [300]: there are good lashes on the upper lid but only a few soft lanugo hairs on the lower [301]

Occasionally ectodermal dysplasia is part of a constellation of defects e.g. prolific Hay–Wells AEC syndrome [106].

'Movie lashes' (trichomegaly) [302], so-called, are long, sparse and luxuriant, the eybrows too. These were recorded because of our love of beauty; it came as a surprise to learn that in very rare instances they have been associated with mental handicap, short stature and pigmentary degeneration of the retina in small-for-dates babies.

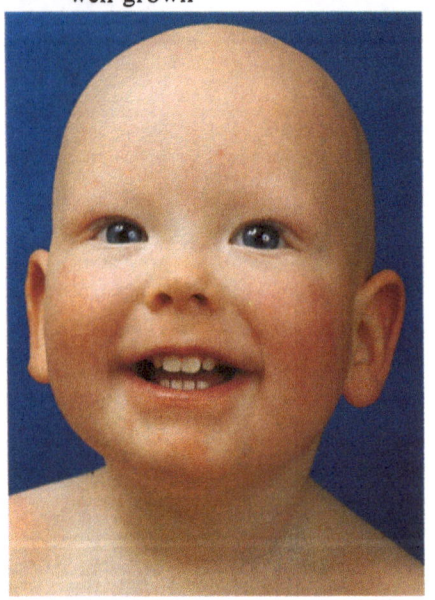

300 Familial ectodermal dysplasia with alopecia totalis . . .

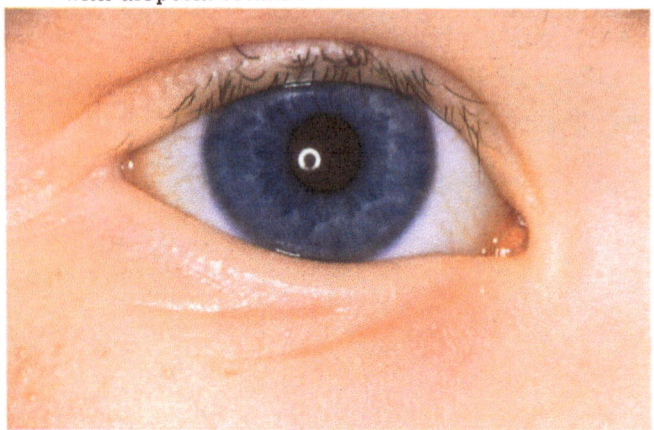

301 In close up one sees that the lower lid has only a few straggly fine hairs of a lanugo variety

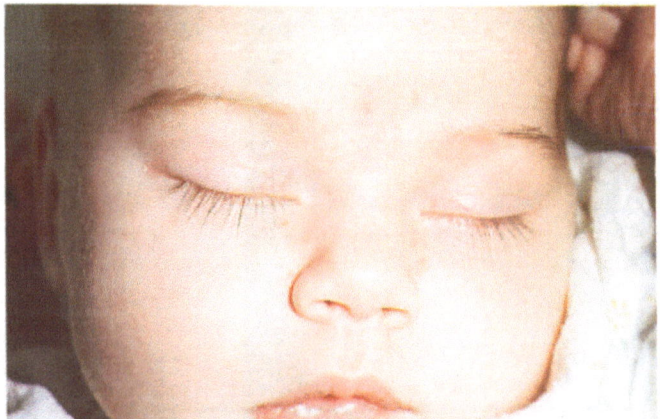

302 9th day

FACIAL MALFORMATION SYNDROMES

'Все взаймосвязано'

'Everything is connected to everything else'

Vladimir Ilyich Ulyanov (Lenin)

Craniofacial dysostosis

Craniofacial dysostosis of the well-known Crouzon or related Saethre-Chotzen type is readily recognized in the nursery; in the florid form [303] there is proptosis because of the shallow orbits, there is antimongolian slant with divergent squint, the nose is beaked and the skull tall. If craniostenosis develops the interval to successful neurosurgical relief is not more than a few weeks [304]. It happened that a favourite 'Crouzon' followed assiduously from birth [305] was correctly reassigned Saethre-Chotzen by a visitor from out of town with slides (Robert Gorlin); minor stigmas differ significantly and characteristically while the management, prognosis and inheritance are similar. In Saethre-Chotzen a prominent ear crus [306] extends across the concha from the root of the helix, there is soft tissue syndactyly [307] index/middle finger, simian crease [308], short little finger and disorders of dermatoglyphics. With severe proptosis [309] divergent strabismus is common.

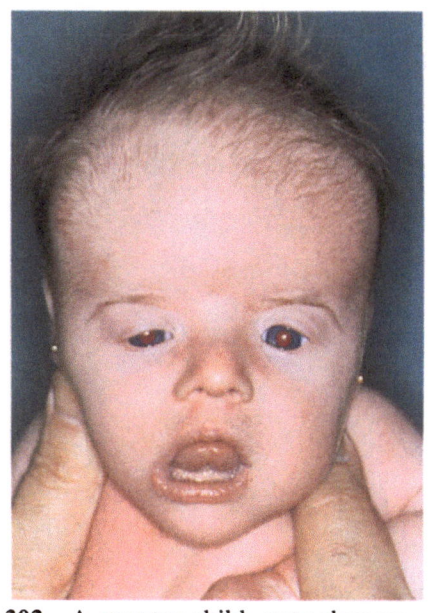

303 A country child, note sleepers

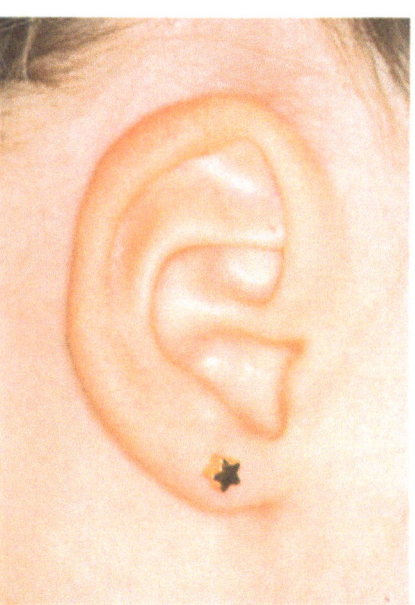

306 Transverse bar

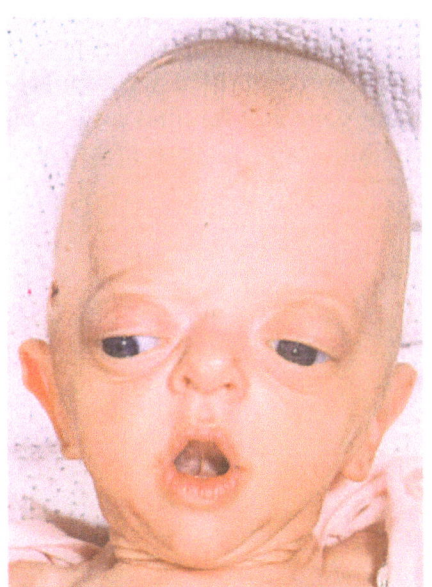

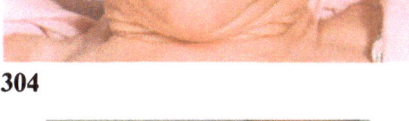

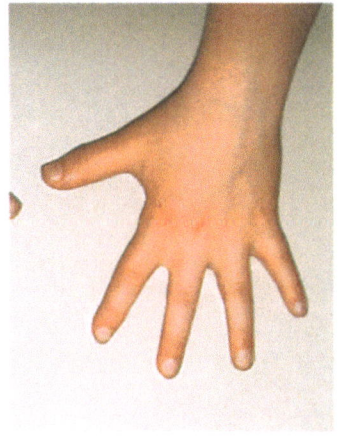

304

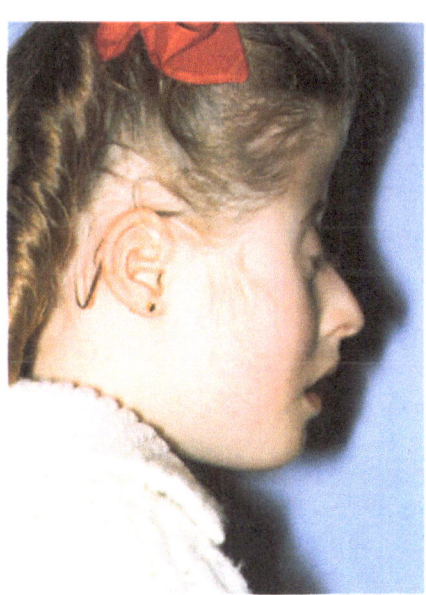

305

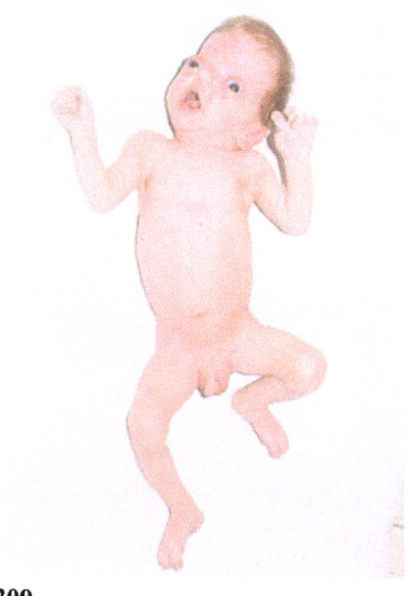

307 Soft tissue syndactyly **308** Simian crease **309**

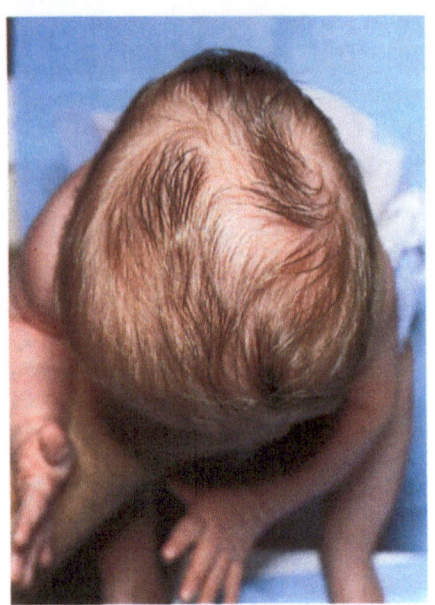

310

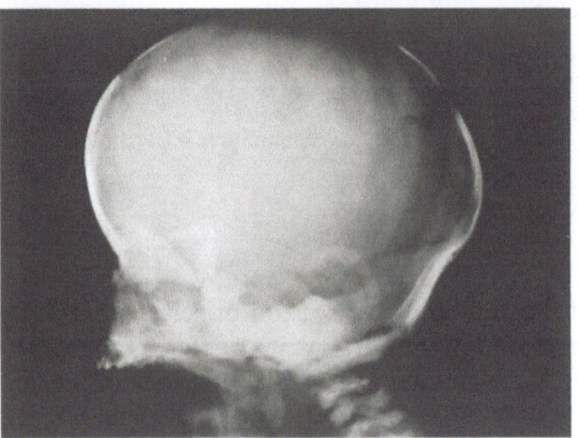

311 Fourth day, early coronal fusion

In this Saethre–Chotzen baby a sutural disorder had caused trigono-cephaly [**310, and see 387, 388**]. Skull X-ray at 4 days [**311**] showed early coronal fusion; a fortnight later this was much worse and acrocephaly was developing, so an operation was done to create new sutures [**312**] and relieve this craniostenosis. Expert opinion proposes that this has been the commonest heritable disorder in which coronal craniostenosis may be an associated feature. The outcome was excellent [**313**] but the nose is more parrot-beak than the averge Crouzon. At 5 years she is in ordinary school and her appearance is not very remarkable, but late plastic surgery is a distinct possibility. Her brother [**314**] also carries the dominant gene that both children inherited from their father [**315**]; this wide variability of clinical expression is typical. Saethre–Chotzen is subtitled acrocephaly-syndactyly type III. Crouzon is a dominant gene and familial cases may occur [**315A, 315B**] with variable expression; about 25 percent of cases represent a mutation.

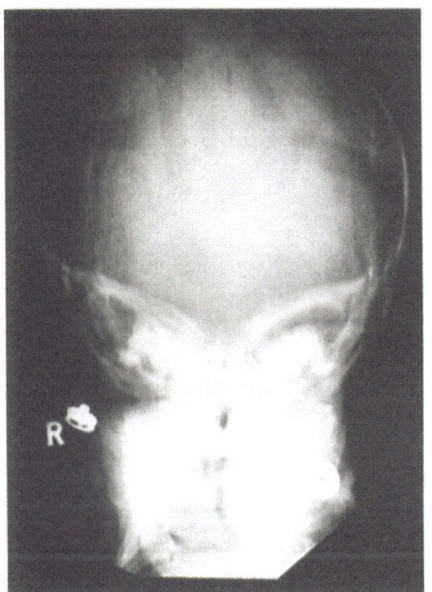

312 Age 3 months, after surgery

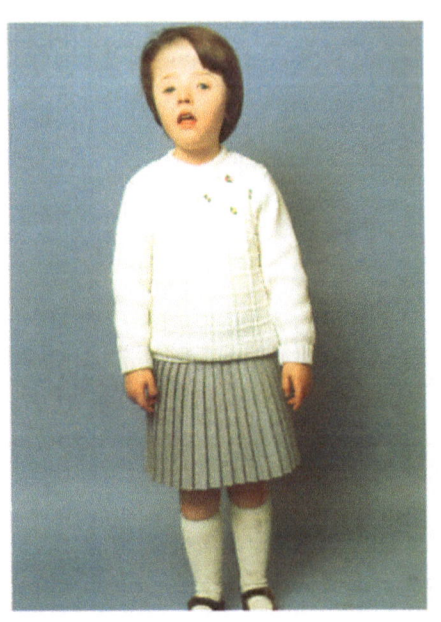

313

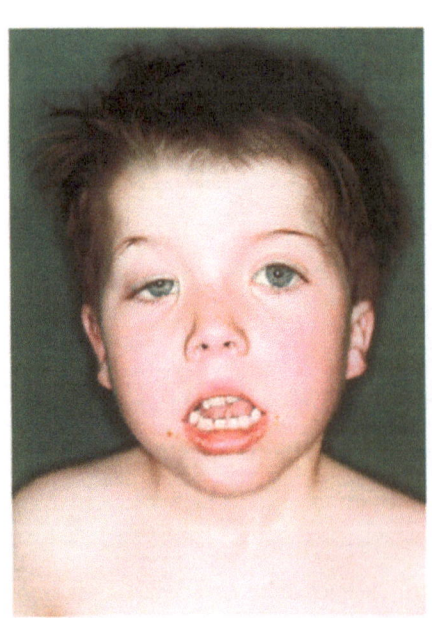

314 Patient's brother . . .

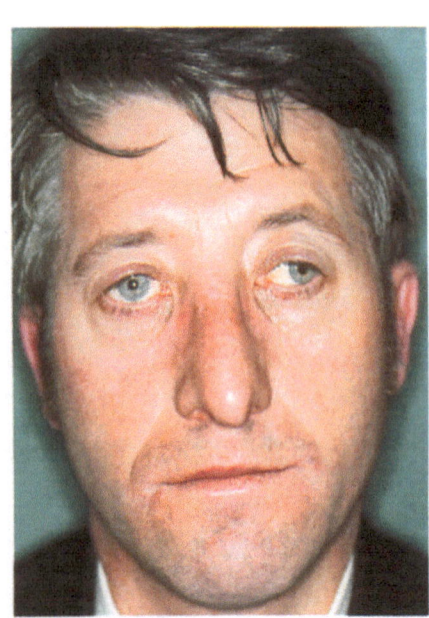

315 And father

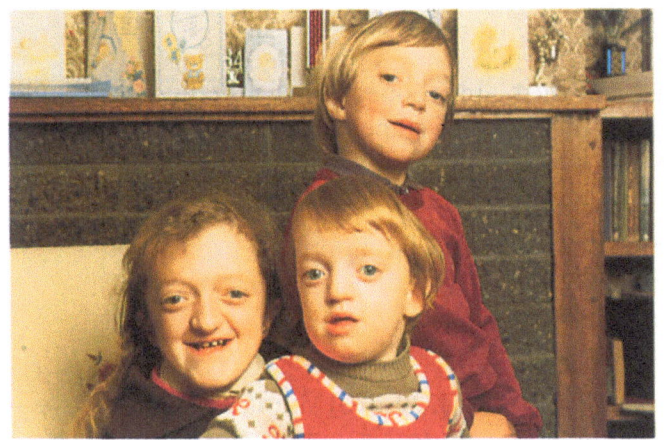

315A

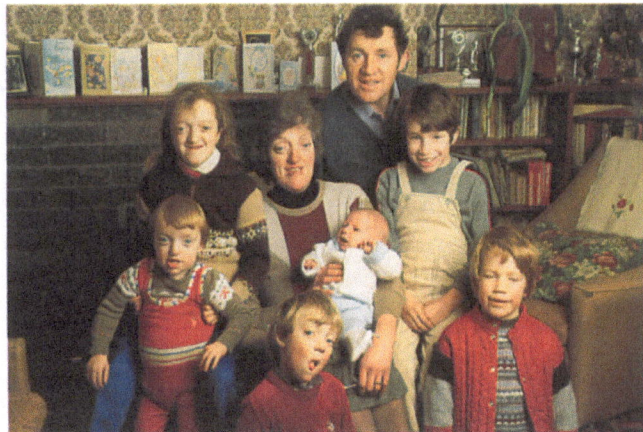

315B

In some cases advanced acrocephaly [**316, 317**], 'tower skull', has already developed *in utero*. On a rare occasion, severe proptosis requires tarsorrhaphy [**113**], to protect the cornea.

Apert acrocephalysyndactyly is similar – roughly speaking it is Crouzon *plus* syndactyly [**318**], *plus* a liability to non-skeletal malformations [**317**].

Carpenter's syndrome presents with acrocephaly and polysyndactyly [**319**], which has led to confusion with Apert's syndrome. The eye changes show some difference: telecanthus and shallow supraorbital ridges are the rule. The main distinction is skeletal: the preaxial polydactyly-syndactyly of the feet. As the survivor grows older there is mental handicap with obesity; this provides scope for confusion with *Lawrence–Moon–Biedl syndrome*.

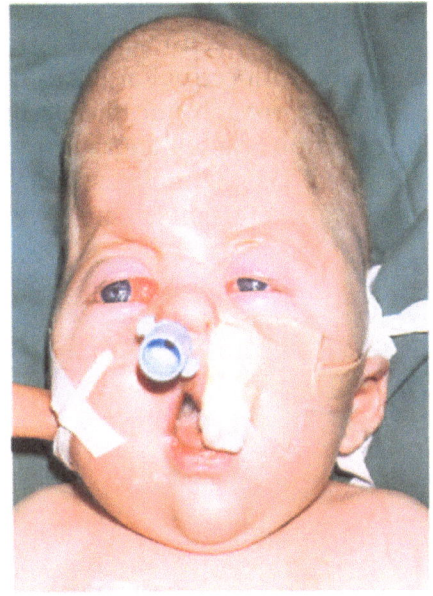

316

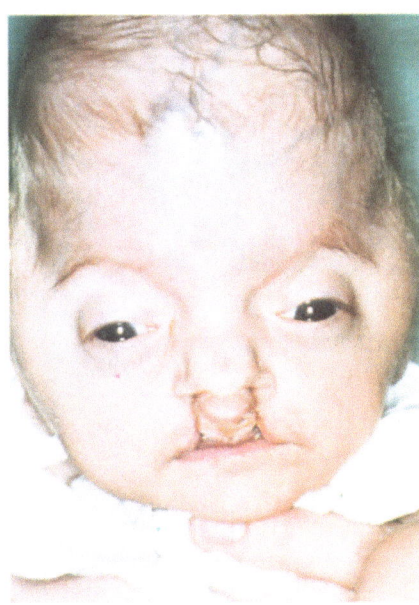

317   Clefts . . . commoner in Apert

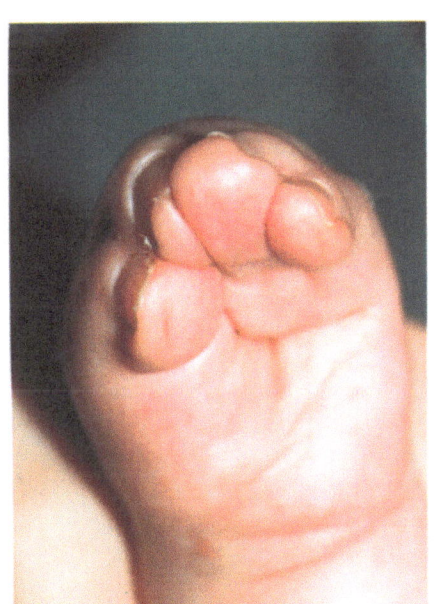

318   Syndactyly

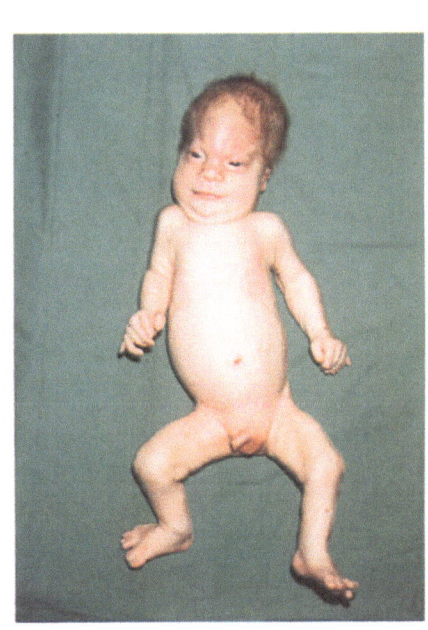

319   Age 5 weeks

First arch syndromes

First arch syndromes, so-called, are grouped together because they could have a common origin in disorders of stapedial artery circulation during embryogenesis; it is the artery of the first branchial arch.

The main ones are:

(1) Treacher Collins mandibulofacial dysostosis
(2) Waardenburg syndrome
(3) Hemifacial microsomia
(4) Goldenhar syndrome

Treacher Collins in this neonate [320–323] shows mandibular hypoplasia, squint, telecanthus, macrostomia, macroglossia and severe deformity of the external ears with tags on the cheeks. There is often hypertelorism with antimongolian slant and the fissures may be short [324]. The usual constellation of facial stigmas is completed by lower lid coloboma with ectropion [325]; here, corneal clouding in the 6 o'clock position is probably due to exposure, the small dense dot in the centre of the left pupil is an anterior cataract. There is also a wide 'V' cleft of the soft palate [326]. A mild case has been shown [286]; extreme variability of clinical expression is notorious. Normal intelligence is the rule, early

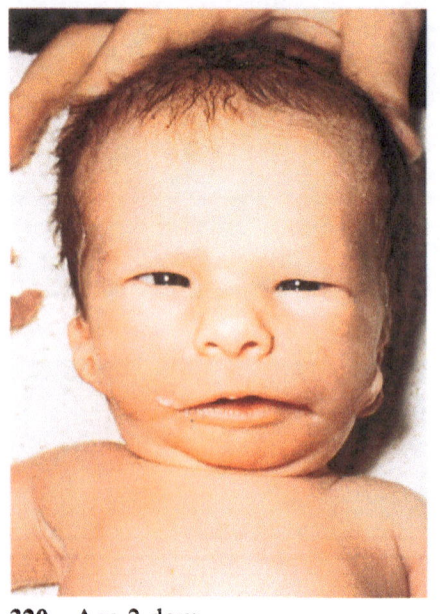

320   Age 2 days

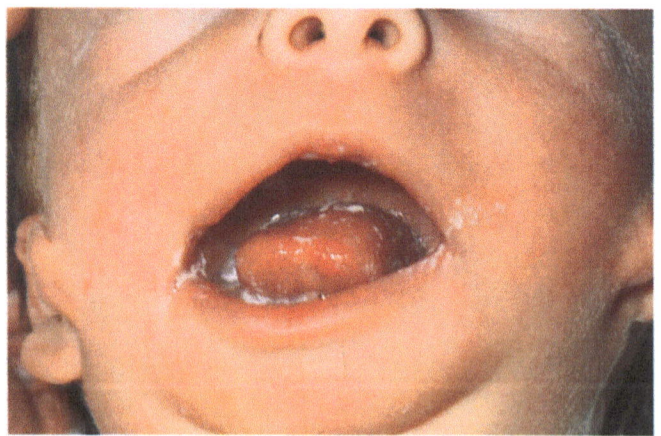

321   Macrostomia

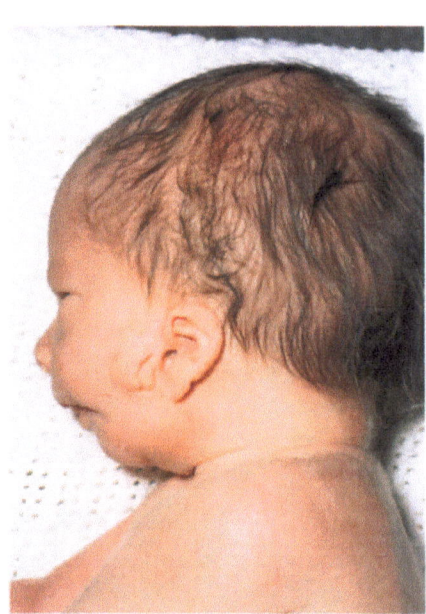

322   Micrognathos

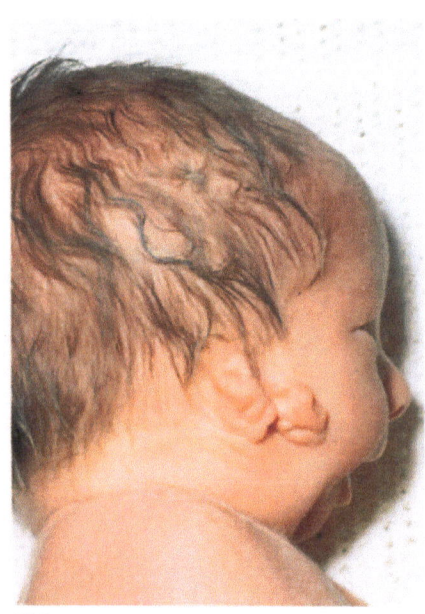

323

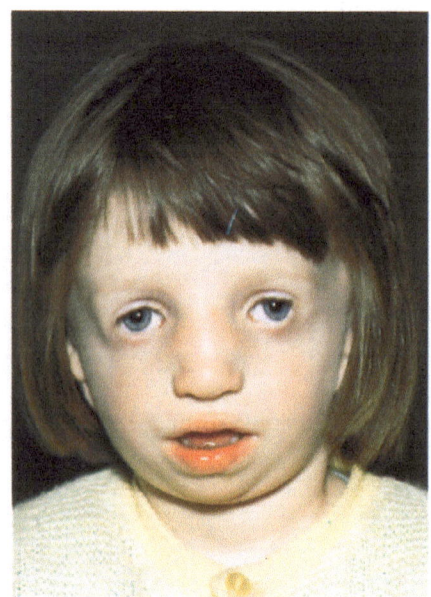

324

otological and plastic surgery opinion is essential because there is often correctable deafness. Inheritance is autosomal dominant, 60% of the cases represent fresh mutations. Affected siblings have a moderate resemblance [327] but the affected parent may have only minimal stigmas; this father carries the gene, so *he is a case, not a carrier*. Sophisticated radiology of mid-face and mandible may give further confirmation of his diagnosis; it is more important to test for conductive deafness and have an ophthalmological opinion. Varients with limb reduction deformities ('acrofacial') have been described; in *Miller's* (postaxial) *syndrome* [328] the deformity is ulnar, in *Nager's* (preaxial) *syndrome* [329] the trouble is radial.

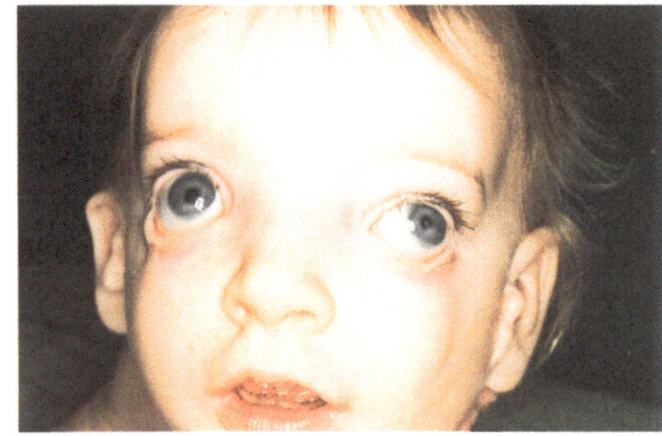

325   Age 1 year

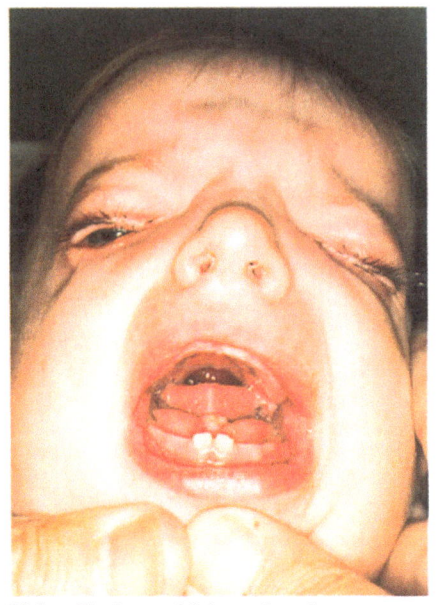

326   Cleft could be missed

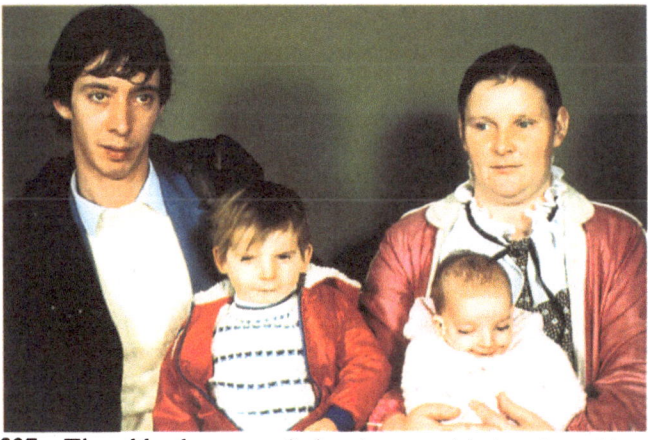

327   The older boy, age 2, has just got his hearing aid; the younger boy wore his from his first birthday

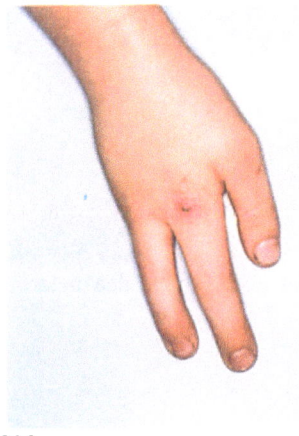

328

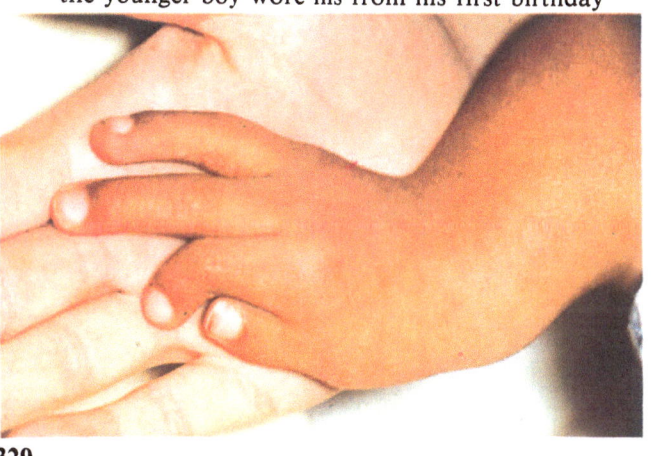

329

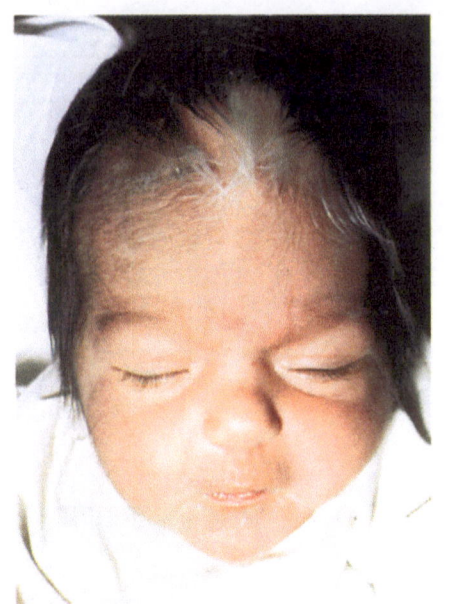

330 Indian baby

Waardenburg is the most exotic, its indicator – the white forelock – may be present at birth [330] but it may not appear until years later. In this case an informed search discovered it because there was a positive family history [331, 332]. The main eye signs are as follows:

Telecanthus occurs due to *dystopia canthorum* (the inner canthi are displaced laterally while the interpupillary distance is normal); this gives a false impression of hypertelorism. Synophrys (fusion of the eyebrows) and heterochromia iris [333] occur, but one suspects that this particular mother could have deleted both the forelock and synophrys. All of the foregoing is merely social or cosmetic; the clinical importance of Waardenburg is that 30% are deaf [334] but normal intelligence is the

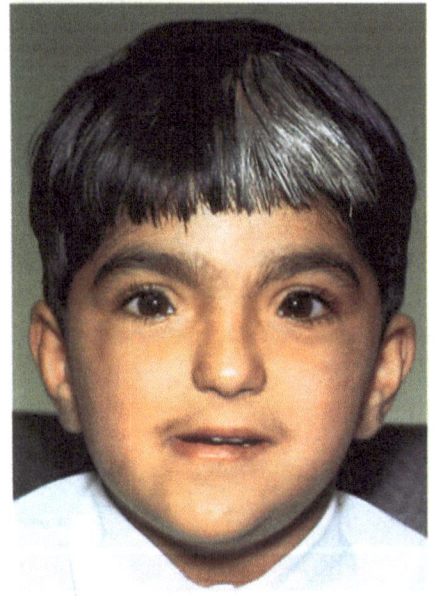

331 Proband

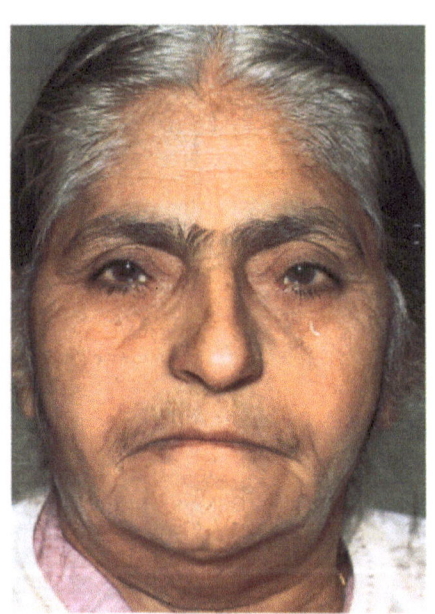

332 Paternal grandmother, father declines to pose

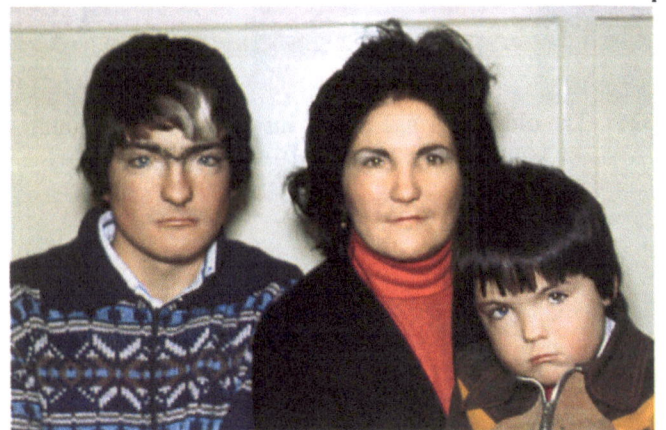

333

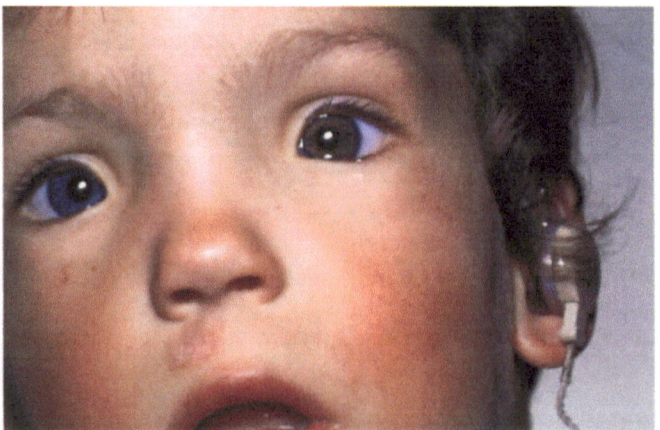

334 30% have deafness

rule. The earlier the child is diagnosed the better [335]; ready acceptance of the hearing aid may give a better outcome than in the late diagnosed older cousin [336] in this pair. The white forelock itself is a trivial form of partial albinism, commonly seen as an isolated defect [337, 338]; it may occur in siblings [339] and the occasional strikingly blue eye colour [334] derives from it. In one bizarre instance a lesion similar to 338 turned out to be an 'achromic naevus' [340] heralding tuberous sclerosis in a child with infantile spasms.

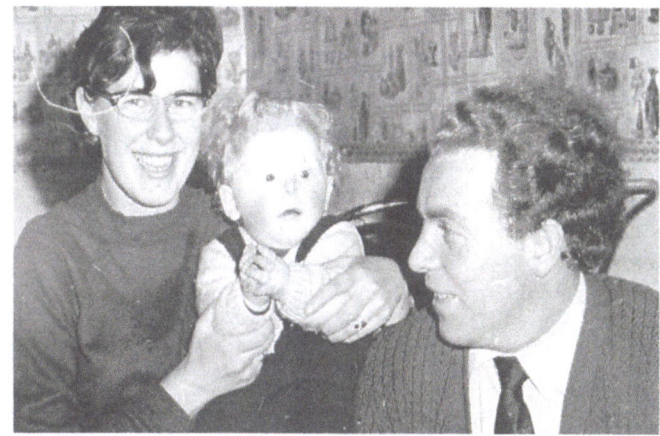

335 Short fissures, prominent alar notching; 11 months

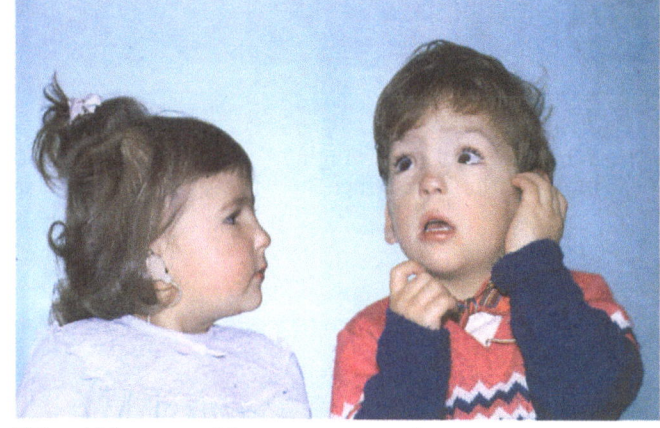

336 Aid accepted by younger cousin

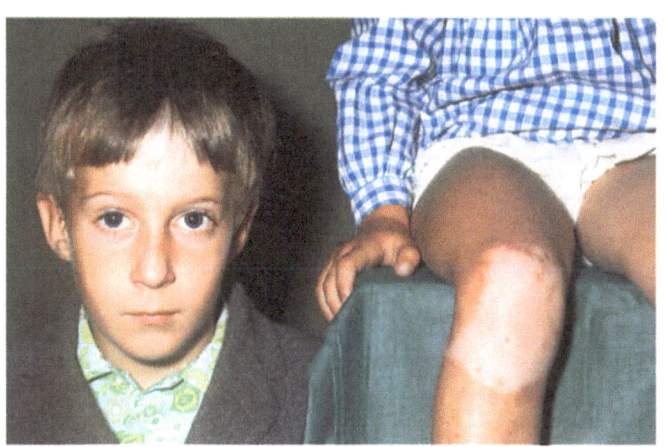

337 Note brilliant blue eyes

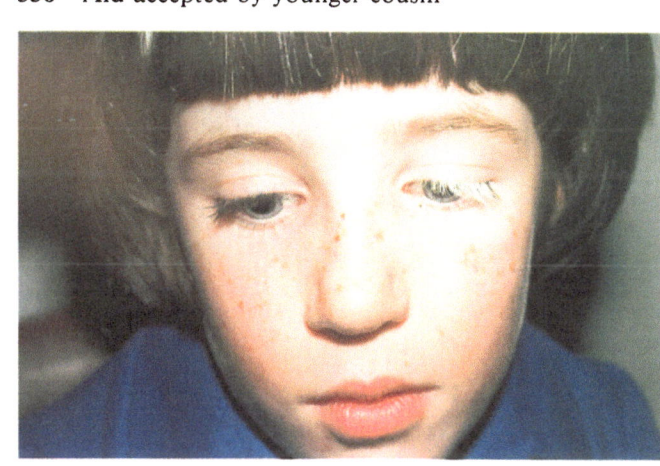

338 Age 7 years

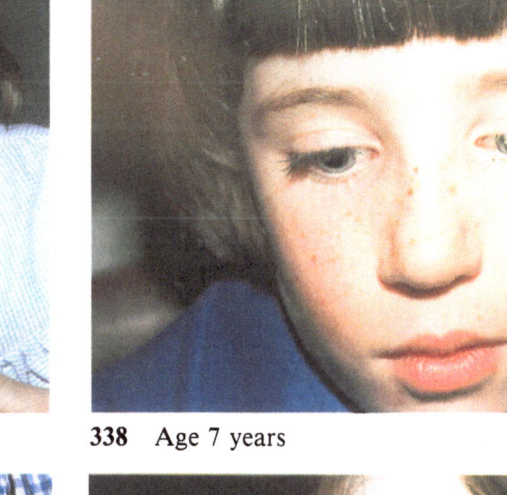

339

340 Depigmentation of eyelashes on the right side, the child developed infantile spasms. Note the fine granular rash of adenoma subaceum on the muzzle are points to the diagnosis of tuberous sclerosis

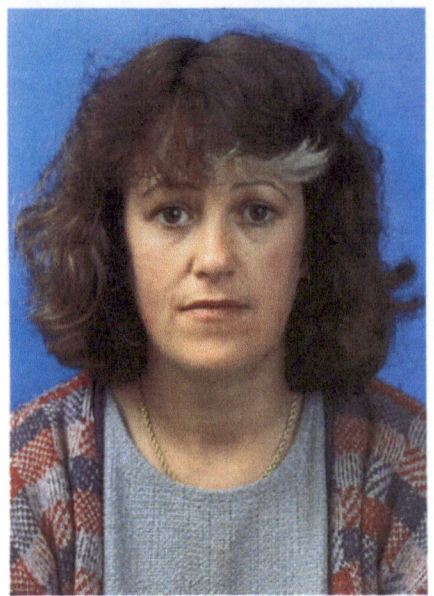

341 White forelock following a blow on the head at age 3

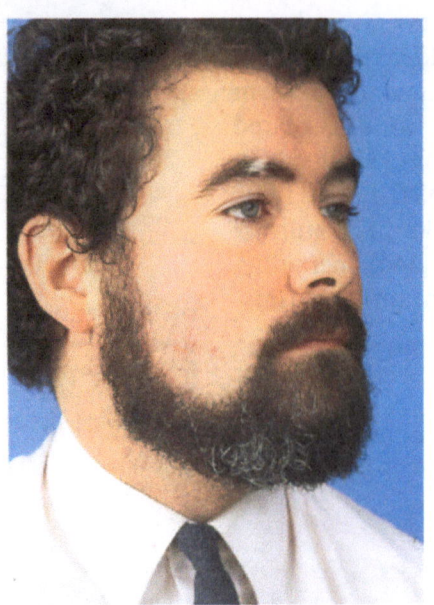

342 Depigmentation following chemical splash in adolescence

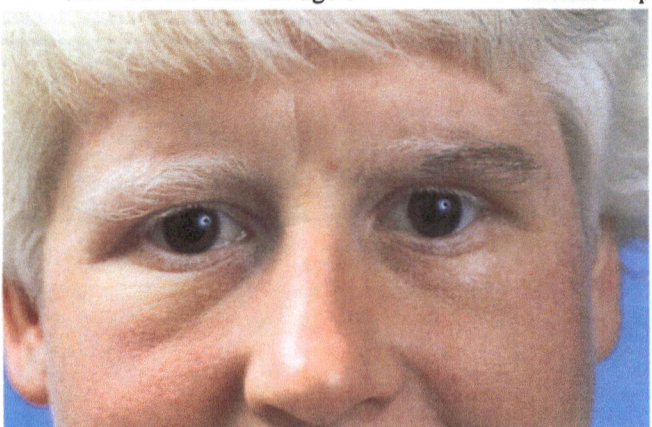

White forelock has been acquired from trauma, a fall on the head at 3 years [341], chemical splashing in adolescence [342]. The converse dark forelock [203] is easily overlooked; note the brilliant blue eye colour. A women with cutaneous albinism had more obvious congenital partial melanism [343] in one eyebrow and the lower eyelashes. Finally, Waardenburg is not confined to man alone [344]. In a referral centre it is inevitable that sooner or later a deaf child with white forelock [345] would prove *not* to be Waardenburg.

343

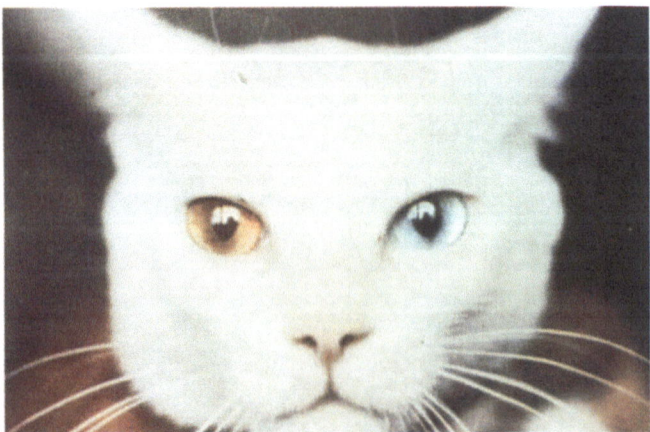

344 First description 1769, this albino cat is at risk of deafness

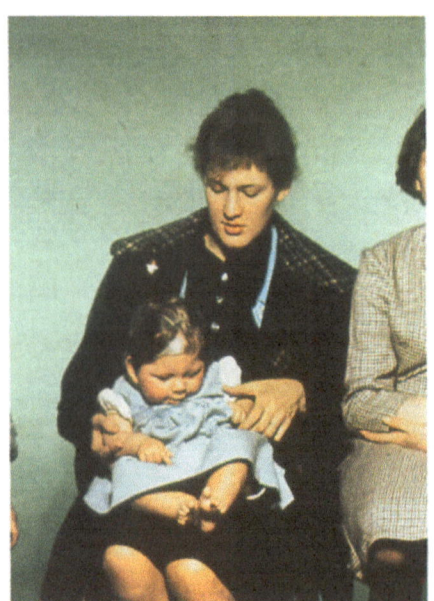

345 Deaf baby with coincidental white forelock; this is *not* Waardenberg

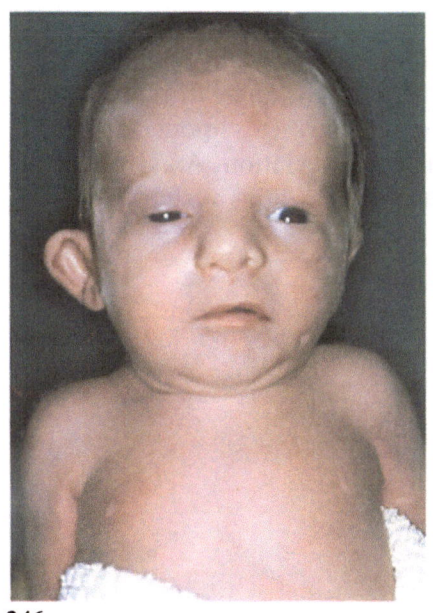

346

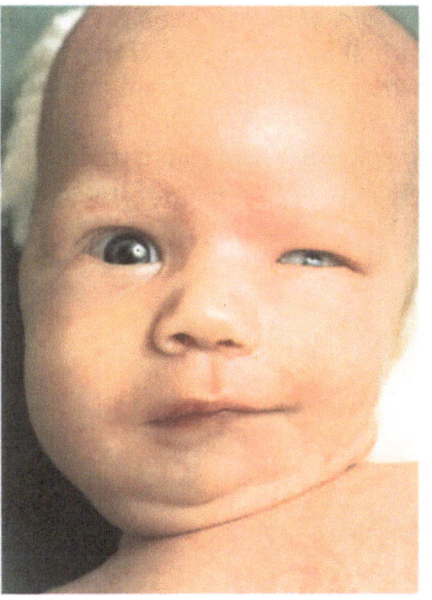

347

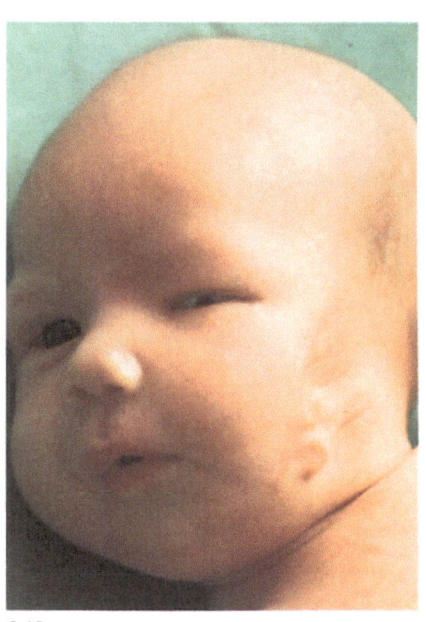

348

Hemifacial microsomia is comparatively straightforward; a relatively mild case [346] shows unilateral facial hypoplasia with microphthalmos, ptosis and 7th nerve palsy with its indicator of 'simple' everted pinna. In a severe case [347, 348] there is marked microphthalmos and extreme malformation of the external ear. Most patients are of normal intelligence, but microphthalmos points to greater risk of mental handicap. It happens to be the syndrome most likely to be associated with upper lid coloboma [348A] here seen in isolation [348B] and of appropriately cautionary subtlety.

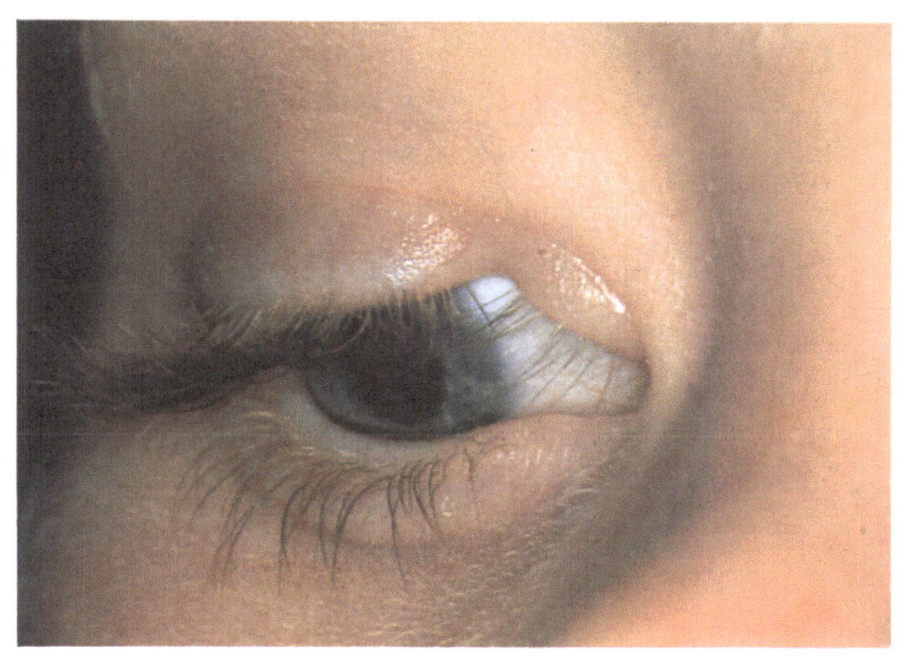

348A

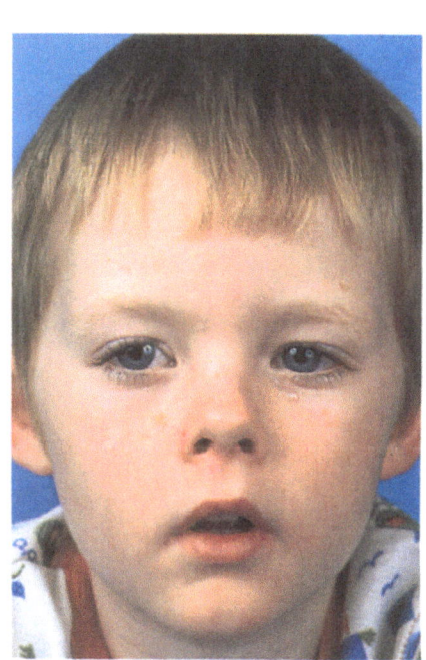

348B

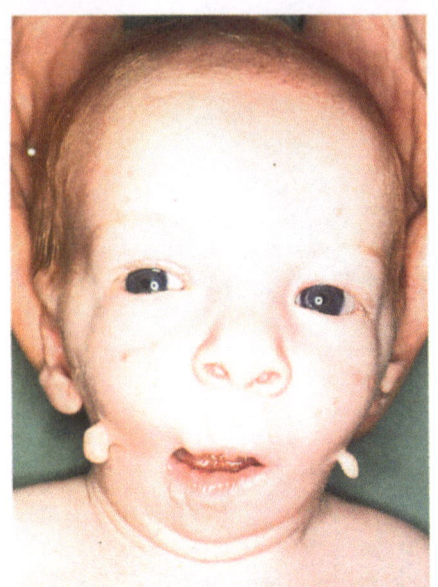

349   Age 1 year

Goldenhar syndrome is very similar [349]; the mandibular hypoplasia with skin tags, hypertelorism with antimongolian slant and squint are prominent. The skin tags are on the line from the angle of the mouth to the auditory meatus [350]. An informed search reveals lipodermoid [351] or epibulbar dermoid, a trivial but constant association. An informed X-ray may now reveal [352] occipitalization of the atlas vertebra.

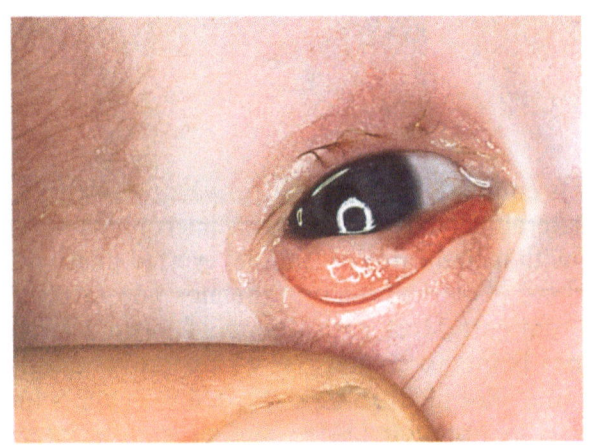

351

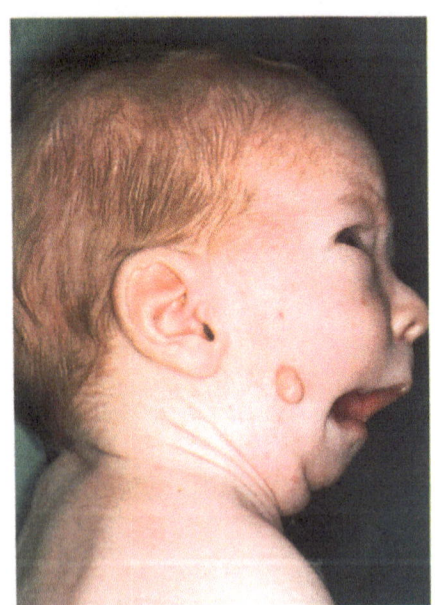

350

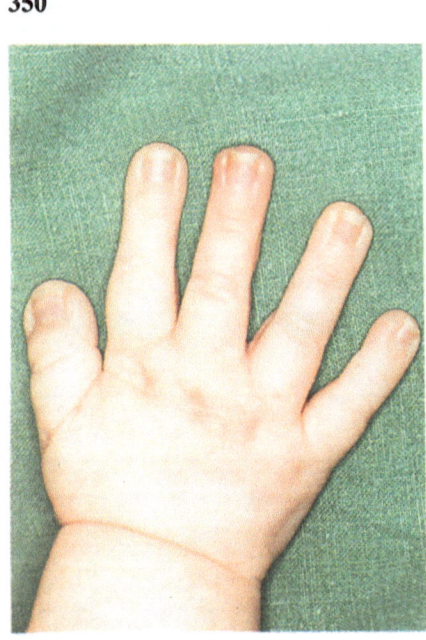

352   Occipitalized atlas

353   354

Rubinstein–Taybi syndrome

Broad thumb and hallux [353, 354] with antimongolian slant and hypoplastic maxilla [355] are the rule, in this case there is ptosis with strabismus and the Marcus Gunn jaw-winking phenomenon occurred [see 94, 95] just to lend variety. Some emphasis has been laid on the variability of the clinical picture, but this would seem to be constant in the facial appearance [356] as compared to the periphery.

Hypertelorism, hypotelorism and midline dysruptive syndromes

The eyes are too far apart or too close-set. Proper centile charts have toppled this last bastion of the subjective school, 'Strong clinical impression, perhaps a touch of hypertelorism. . . .' [357, 358]. The centile readings confer accuracy in their usual way, but it is only 97^+ or 3^- centile readings that are properly significant. The most reliable clinical measurement is the inner canthal, at the inner end of the medial canthus; the outer canthal distance is also measured. If both are 97^+ centile this is *hypertelorism*, if the outer is normal it is *telecanthus*. In telecanthus the inner canthi have moved laterally, *dystopia canthorum*; the amount of sclera showing is reduced. The most significant X-ray measurement is the *inner orbital* but it does not have much to add in the average case. It is not surprising that hypertelorism and hypotelorism commonly feature in a number of syndromes of midline dysruption and when they are a prominent stigma then the possibility of these syndromes must be kept in mind.

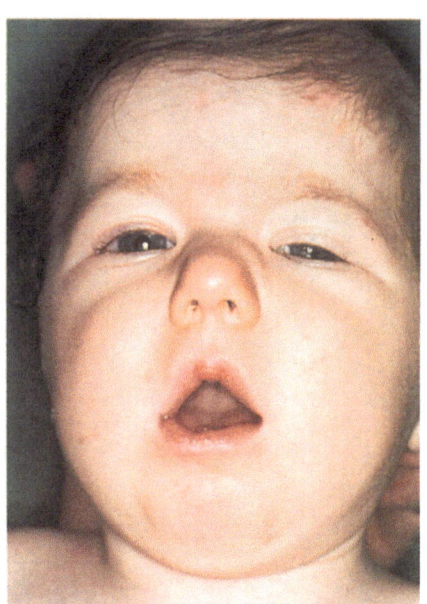

355 Age 5 months

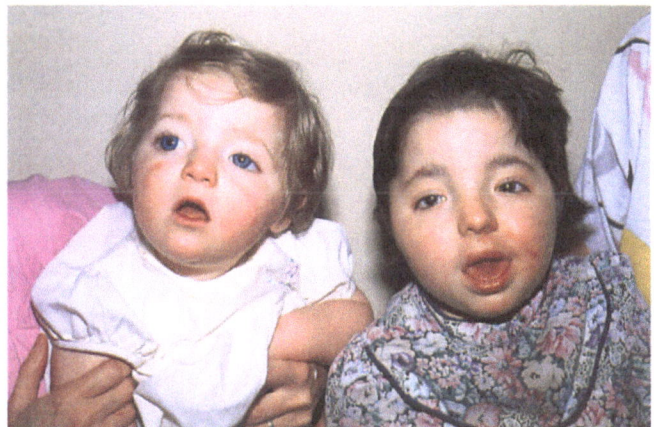

356 Two unrelated cases

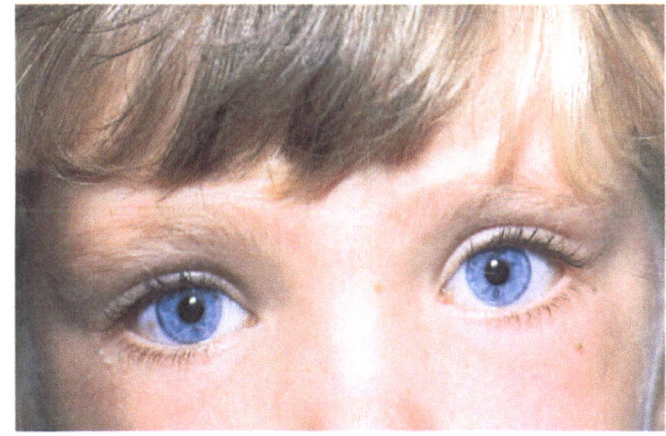

357 Clinical impression of hypertelorism, 5 years old

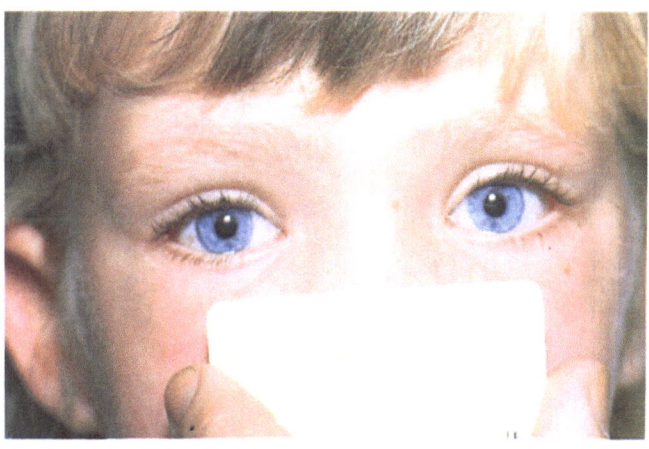

358 Inner canthal distance 31 mm, interpapillary 53 mm, both 75th centile

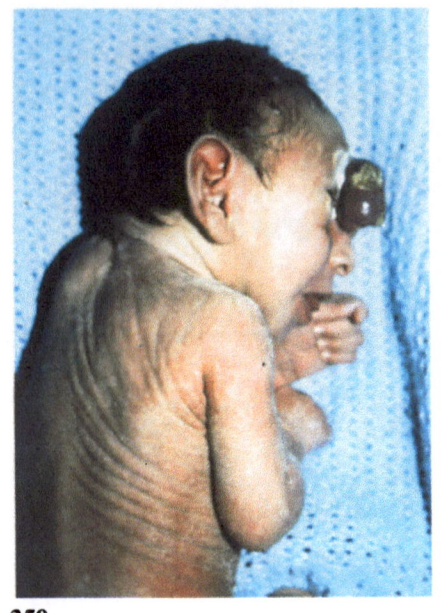

359

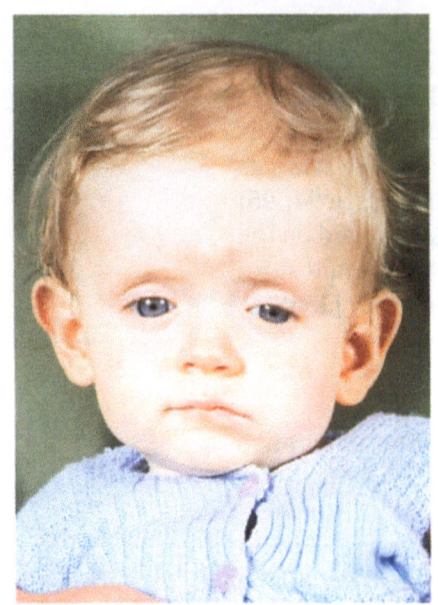

360 Age 1 year

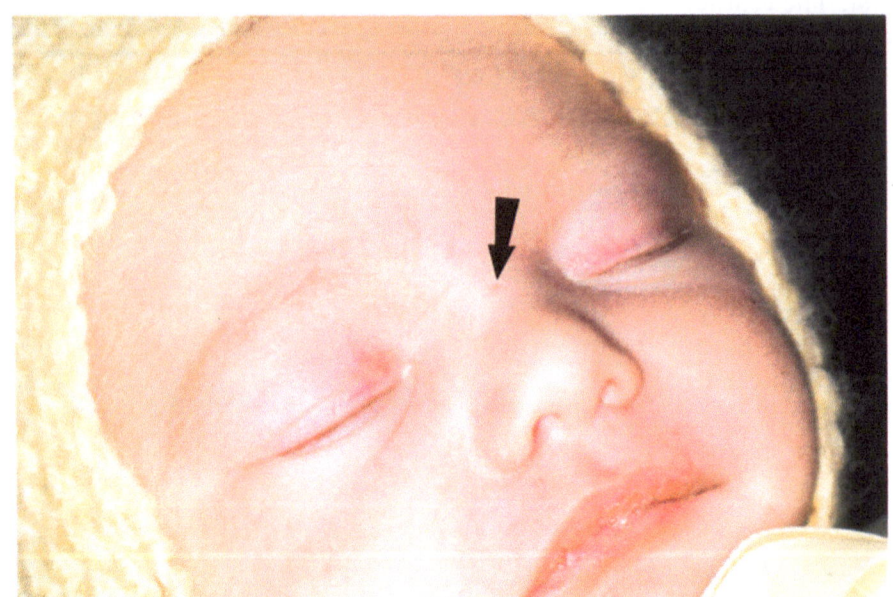

361 In the midline the least . . .

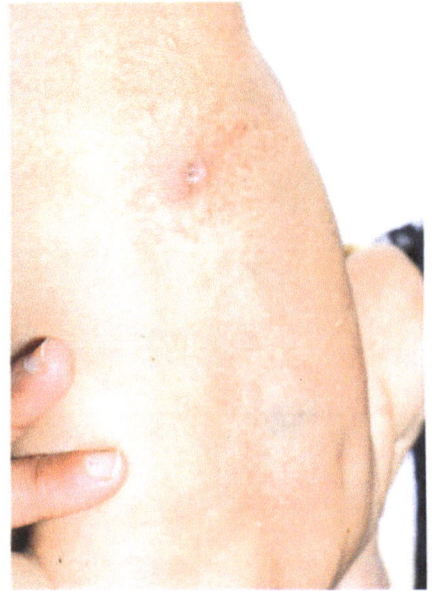

362 . . . Defect always . . .

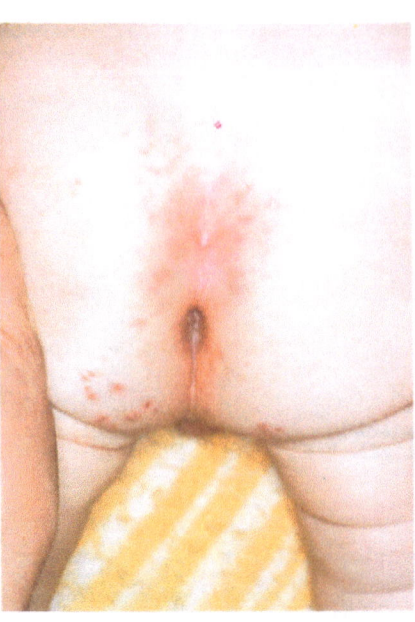

363 . . . Commands the greatest respect

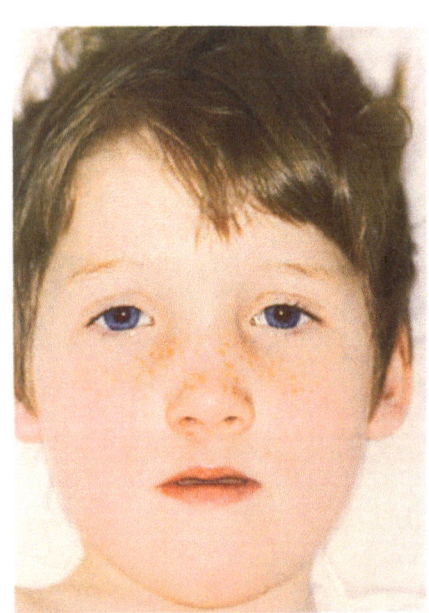

364

Hypertelorism with degrees of failed midline fusion is well known. Severe anterior exocephaly [359] in this baby appropriately enough overshadows the hypertelorism almost to the point of invisibility. Even the smallest associated midline swelling [360] is an emergency; it may be the tip of the iceberg. The very tiniest pit [361] is an emergency, since there may be fistula. It is the rule that defects tend to be multiple, so the whole length of the line of midline closure must be inspected minutely [362, 363]. The most subtle lesion of all is concealed, a defect of the cribriform plate [364]. This boy had mild clear discharge from the right nostril since birth (CSF rhinorrhoea). He survived two attacks of meningitis before undergoing surgery at age 3 years.

Hypertelorism is associated in some instances with a degree of midline disruption such as median cleft face [365, 366]. Hypertelorism itself often causes divergent squint [e.g. 372] and facial clefting may aggravate it, but this is not necessarily so [367]. Here one can usefully refer to the facial dysplasia syndromes [303–352], especially Crouzon, Saethre–Chotzen and Waardenburg.

Hypotelorism is characterized by eyes too closely set; the inner canthal distance is below the 3rd centile. It too is usually associated with forms of midline dysruption.

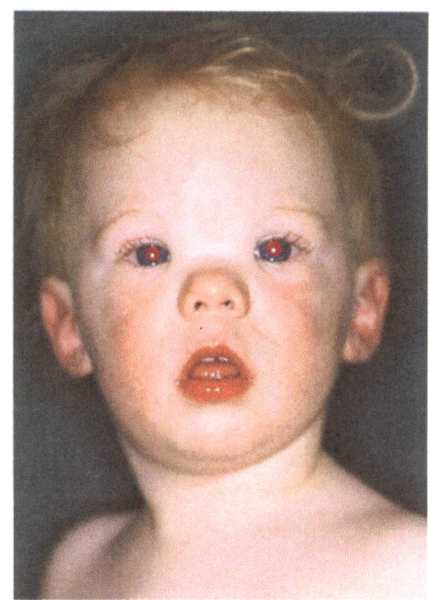

365 Mild . . .

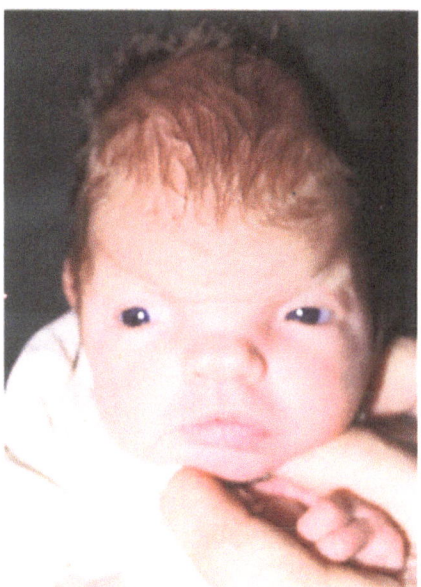

366 Less mild . . .

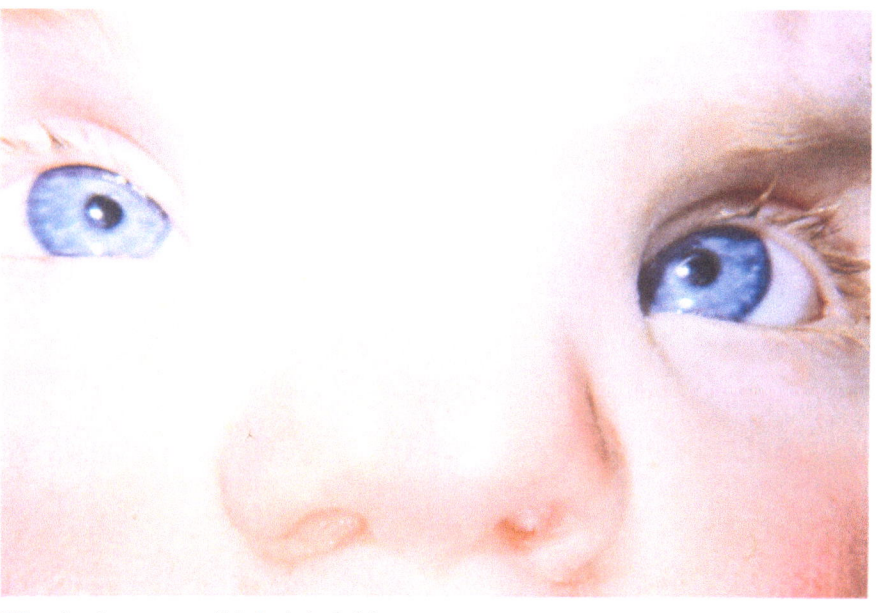

367 And not so mild facial clefting

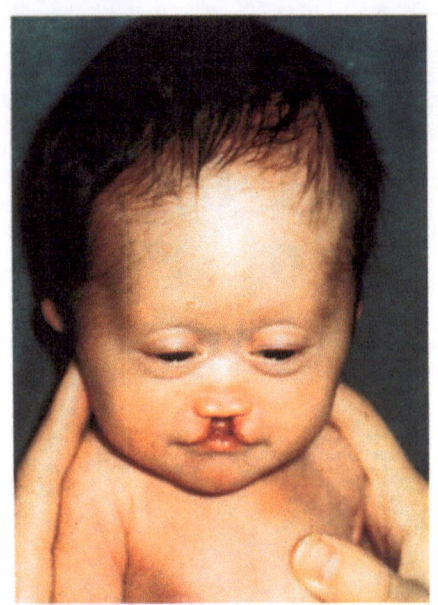

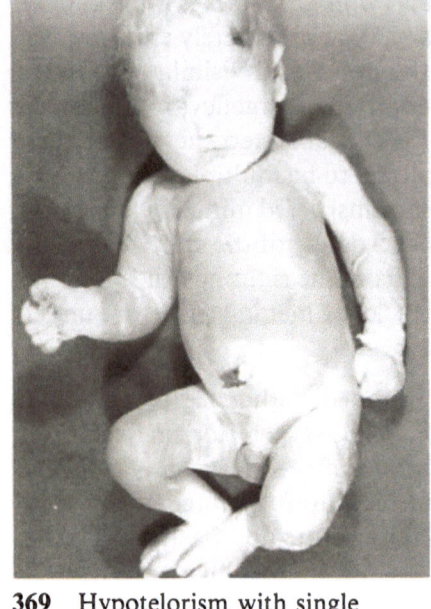

The holoprosencephaly sequence is a rare but well-known cause; there is premaxillary agenesis, flat nose and hypotelorism [368], cebocephaly [369] and cyclopia-synotia [370] among its stages. In advanced forms there is forebrain disruption [371] with single ventricle and absent corpus callosum.

368 Mild

369 Hypotelorism with single nostril, cebocephaly ('monkey face'!). Moderate

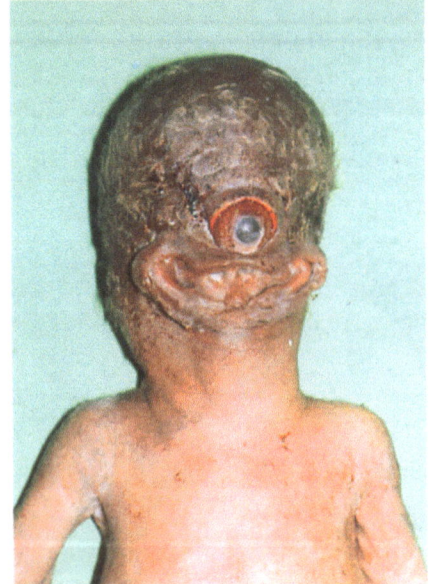

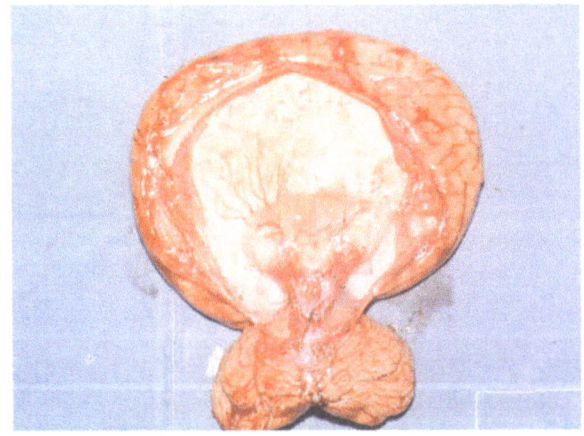

370 Severe

371 Cerebral holosphere, absent septum pellucidum

NEWER MIDLINE DYSRUPTION SYNDROMES
(many with symmetrical stigmas)

Disorders of midline fusion have the distinction of historical primacy combined with an early perception that their common features made it attractive to group them together, separate from but contiguous with the general. The result was a positive constructive step in taxonomy; any fears of a divisive effect were unfounded. In general the historical lesions were more or less obvious, the causative mechanisms appeared clear, and everyone is aware of the two classical snags, first the 'submerged iceberg' element and secondly the genetic dimension common to most of them.

Unfortunately, things are far less rosy with regard to appreciating some of the newer syndromes of midline dysruption, if we consider the waves of discovery that marked the decade following Patau's awesome curtain-raiser in 1960. With a little shuttling between North America and the European landmass some semblance of order may be imposed and at the same time some question marks arise.

Opitz hypertelorism–hypospadias syndrome (1965), officially B-B-B syndrome (original family names Bohnert, Betts, Bryant), 'H–H' syndrome, has *h*ypertelorism [372] and *h*ypospadias [373] as its basis; there are other midline features such as facial clefting [372] and there are symmetrical lesions such as hand deformities [374], congenital inguinal hernia and undescended testicles. The condition is fully expressed in the male but in the female limited to hypertelorism [375], exemplifying autosomal dominant inheritance with partial male sex limitation. *The most important stigma* is dull normal intelligence, the worst form of mental handicap in relation to the child's needs, especially if he looks peculiar – many affected boys were backrow educational sediment, unnecessarily. *Resolve:* the ophthalmologist to enquire about the nether region as appropriate, the perineal surgeons to raise their sights above the symphysis pubis. Every newborn boy with hypospadias and/or undescended testicles and/or inguinal hernia must be seriously considered possibly to have a problem beyond surgery until proved otherwise; this includes early responsible medical referral. Most surgical publications on hypospadias, for instance, are no more than publications on hypospadias and its adjacent Metro suburbia.

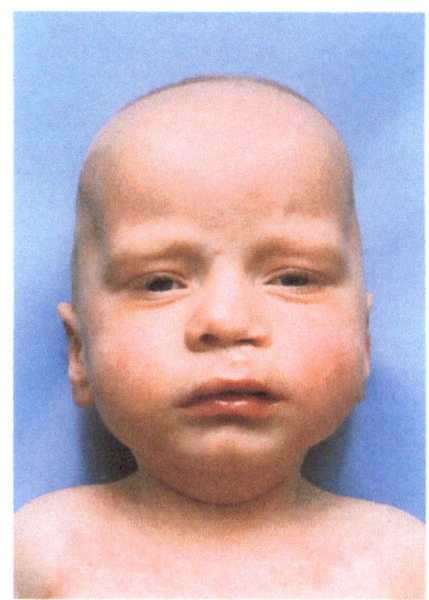

372   Lip repaired

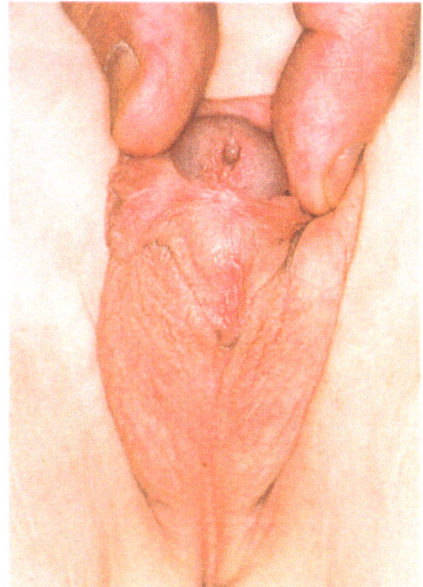

373   Mild hypospadias

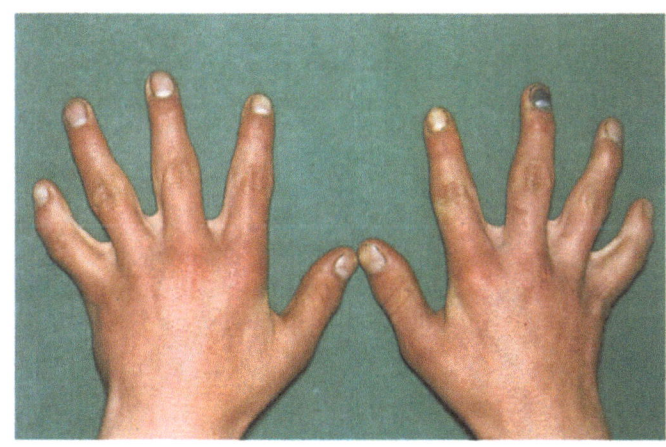

374   Stumpy fingers with webbing

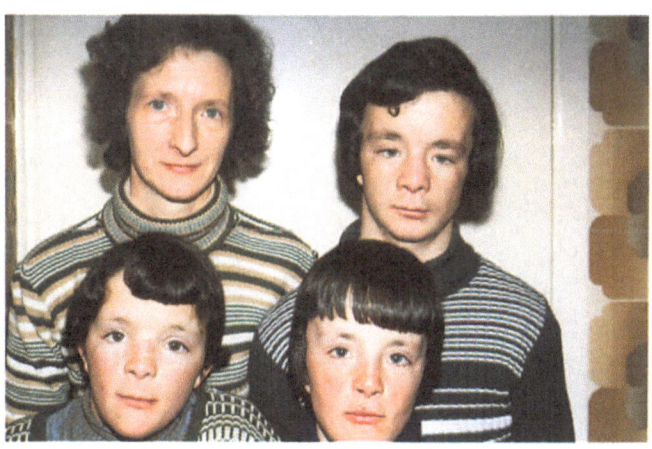

375

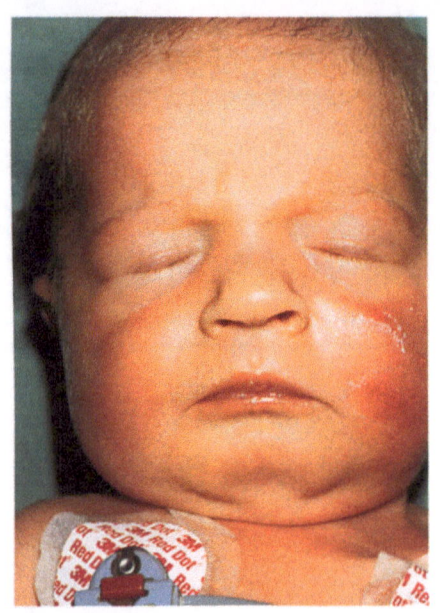

Opitz–Frias(G) syndrome (1969) (original family name: Georgeson) has much in common with the B–B–B syndrome, including inheritance. Typical facial appearance [376] includes hypertelorism of mild to moderate degree and antimongolian slant and here there is a little oedema (associated with patent ductus arteriosus [377]), while fine bubbling at the lips is arising from oesophageal atresia [378] laryngotracheosophageal anomalies being almost invariable. There was anterior anus [379]. The vulva was remarkable, there was 'diastasis' of the labia majora as if the fourchettes had not formed properly, and the labia minora were prominent. Most cases are male; bifid scrotum [380] is the common lesion; one could perhaps think of the girl as having 'bifid vulva' if that is not too paradoxical*.

*Dr Opitz accepts this is a case.

376 Note fine bubbles

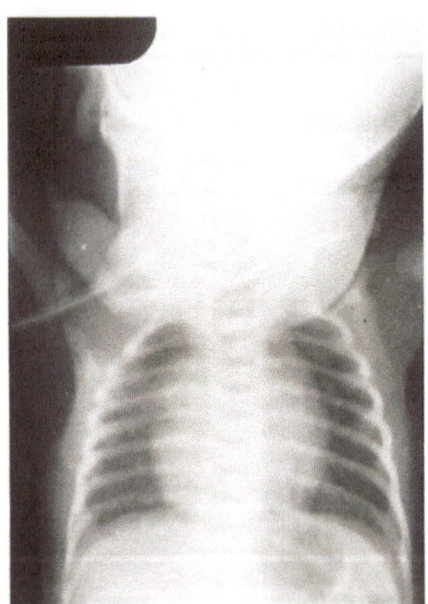

377 Globular heart shape

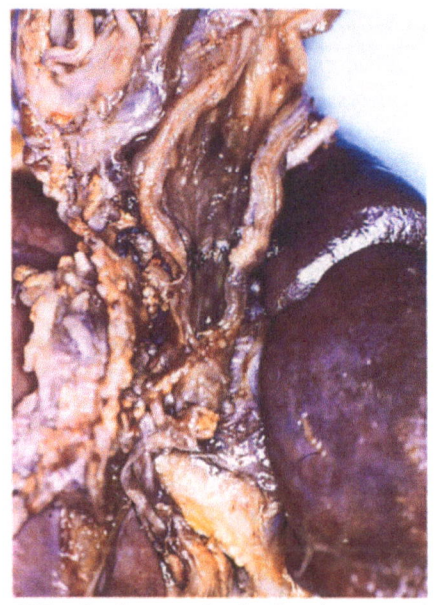

378 Patient expired after intracranial bleed. Note thick hide-like pouch sutured to thin-walled lower segment

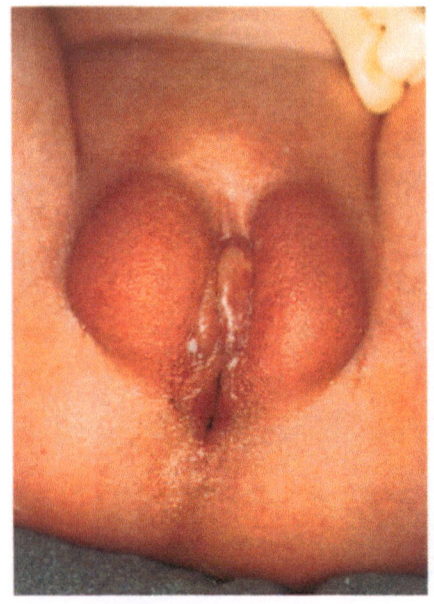

379 'Bifid' vulva, anterior anus

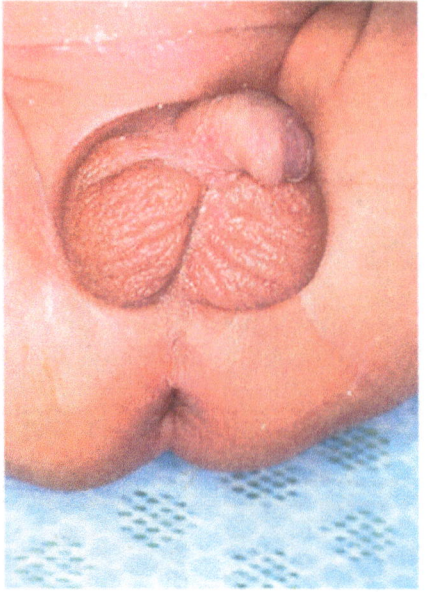

380 Bifid scrotum

In another unclassified 'midline' case severe hypertelorism and metopic suture diastasis [381] was associated with extreme persistent tracheo-malacia and laryngotracheal cleft. His genitalia were normal. A brother was similarly affected [382] and the mother and aunt [383] had hyper-telorism. Time has begun to bring a gratifying amelioration of the facial appearance [384].

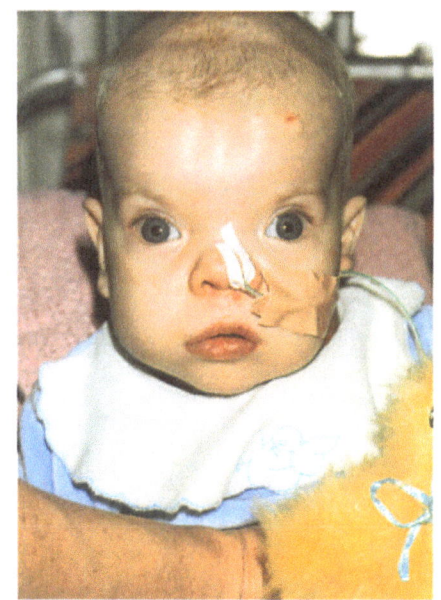

381 Age 5 months

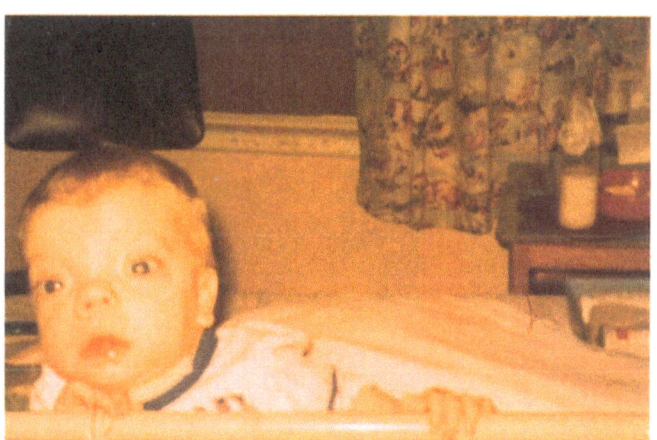

382 Age 7 months

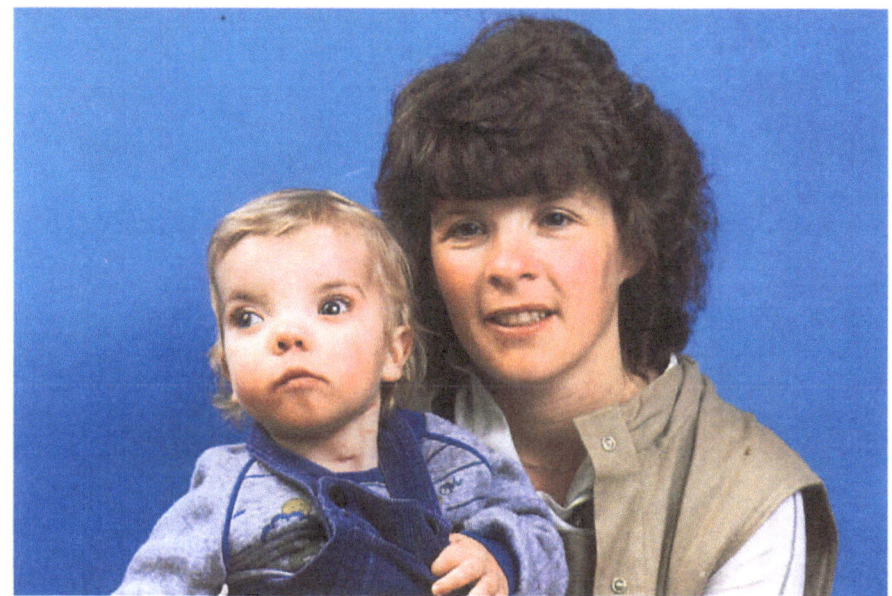

383 Inner canthal distance maternal aunt 38 mm (97$^+$ centile), patient 40 mm

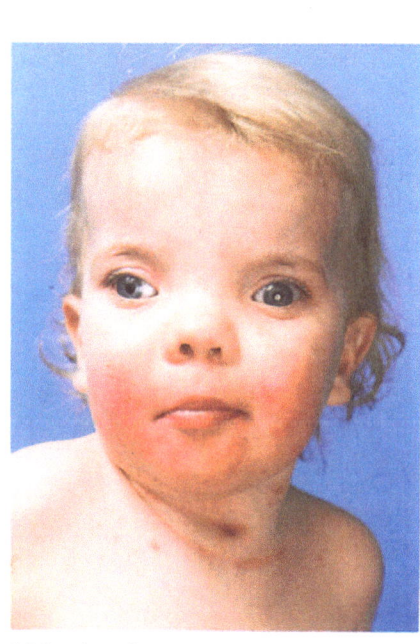

384 Age 2 years

Opitz trigonocephaly (C) syndrome (1969) (original family name: Camus) has premature fusion of the metopic suture causing hypotelorism with a midline ridge [385], broad nose with epicanthus and squint [386], and trigonocephaly. Further features, by an acronymic quirk, are *C*left palate, *C*ongenital heart disease and *C*ryptorchidism.

Isolated metopic suture fusion causes hypotelorism [387] with trigonocephaly [388]; it is harmless. We have already seen another form of trigonocephaly, the reverse of this, in the Saethre–Chotzen disorder [310]; it is potentially dangerous.

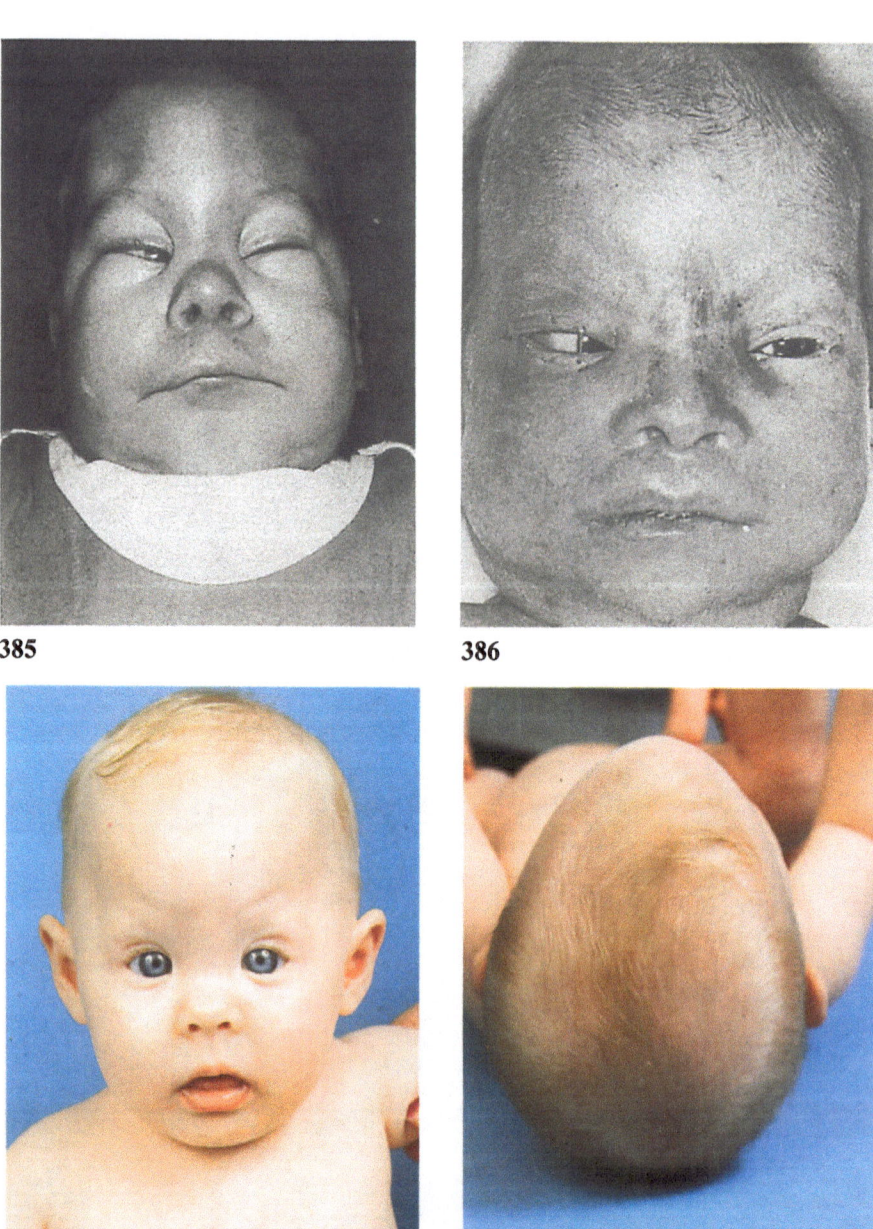

385

386

387   Age 6 months

388

Robinow fetal face syndrome (1969) combines hypertelorism **[389]**, irregular dentition **[390]**, small penis with cryptorchism **[391]** and deep pilonidal dimple **[392]** that may overlie hemivertebra. These illustrations are post-neonatal, a justifiable liberty in view of the *'fetal face'* label that cleverly smuggles it through the routine nursery examinations.

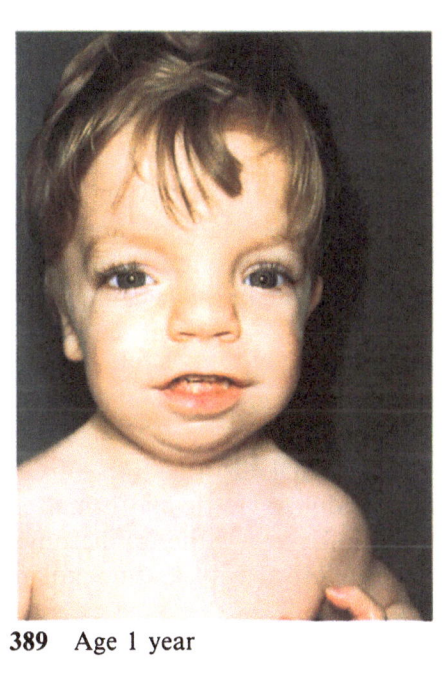

389   Age 1 year

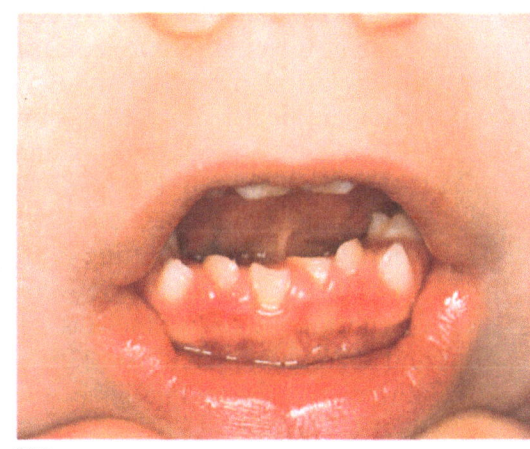

390

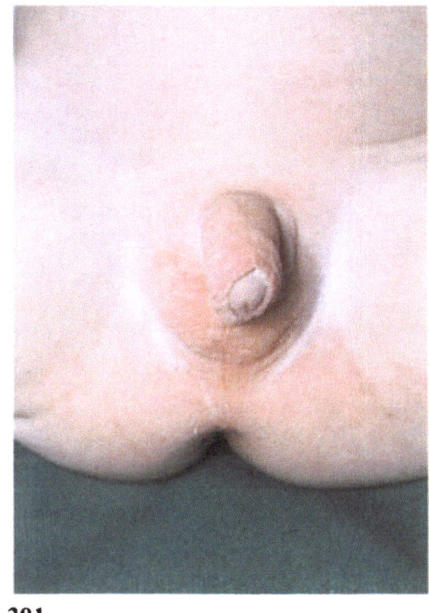

391

392

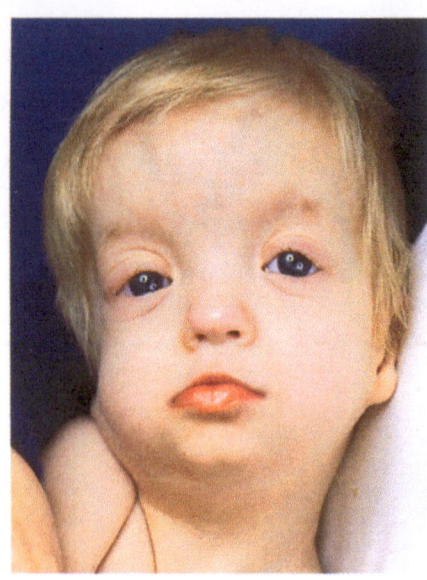

393 Patient with Opitz hypertelorism–hypospadias, the appearance of the mouth would be expected more commonly and characteristically in Aarskog syndrome

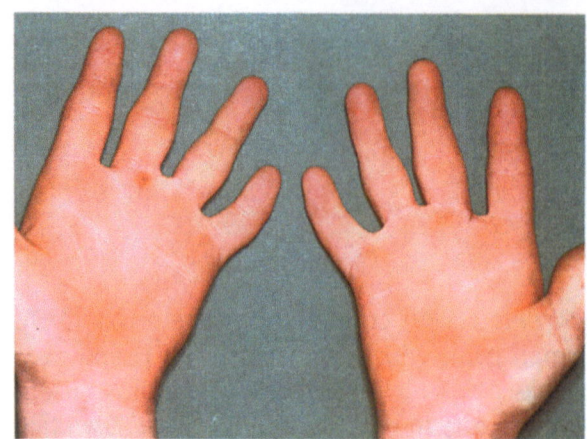

394 Brachydactyly in Opitz hypertelorism–hypospadias syndrome, it is more usually thought of as one of the hall marks of Aarskog syndrome

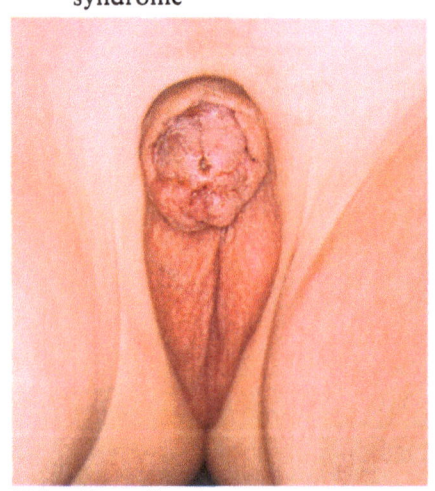

395 'Shawl' scrotum

Aarskog syndrome (1970) has hypertelorism, brachydactyly and shawl scrotum. It would seem to come somewhere between Robinow and Opitz hypertelorism–hypospadias. By their nature, syndromes overlap so although one has not yet recognized a case of Aarskog one can quickly assemble an 'Identikit' by adding to the basic hypertelorism the mouth [393], brachydactyly [394] and shawl scrotum [395] with cryptorchism from similar syndromes. But *true* Aarskog has *intactness*, of intellect, lip, palate, and urethra, putting it beyond this prestidigitation.

Cri-du-chat syndrome reflects a chromosomal disorder (5p−): the diagnosatic kitten-like mewing cry at birth is due to glottic malformation and there is hypertelorism [396]. As the glottis grows the cry becomes normal and the main stigma is then hypertelorism with antimongolian slant [397, 398].

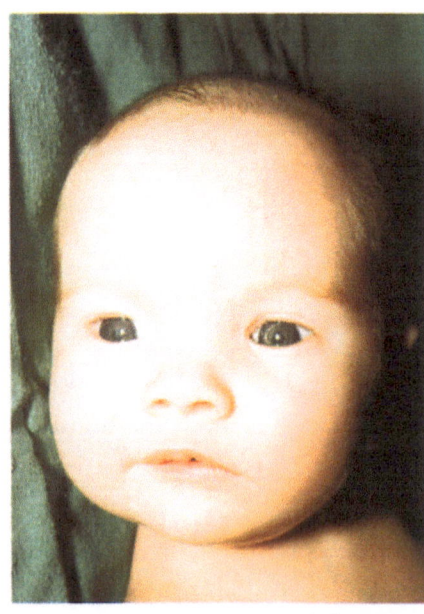

396 Commonly diagnosed from next room

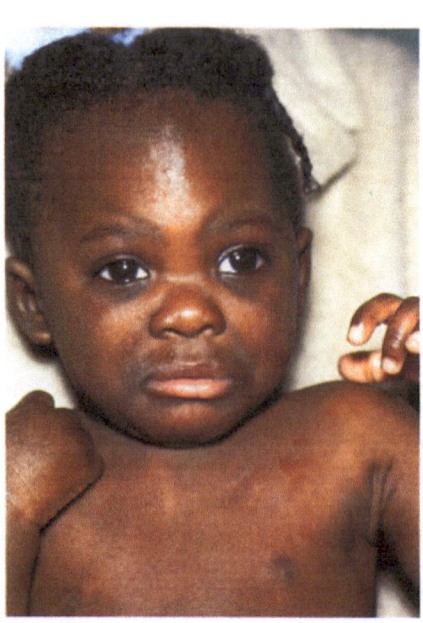

397 Age 2 years

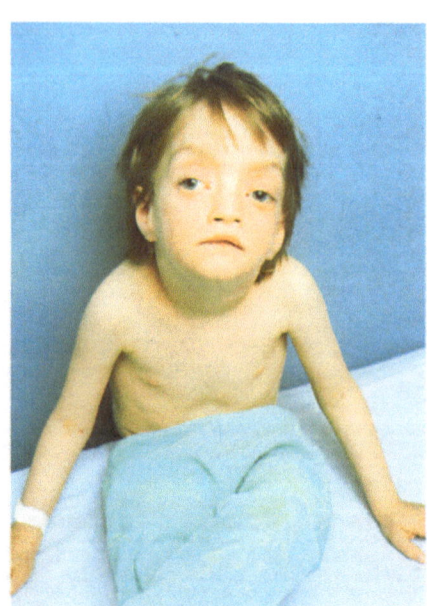

398 Age 7 years

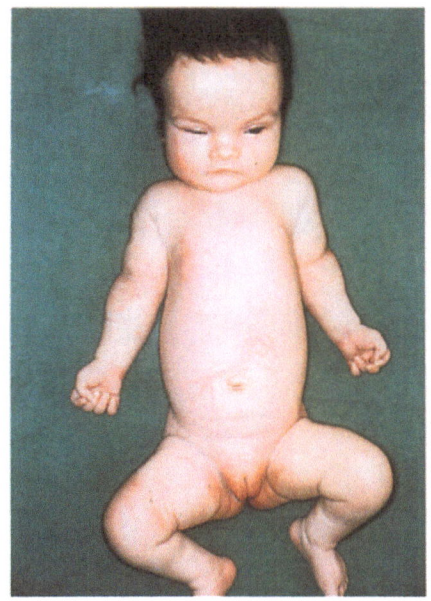

399 Apathy and hypotonia with rather large (40 cm) square shaped head, fisting

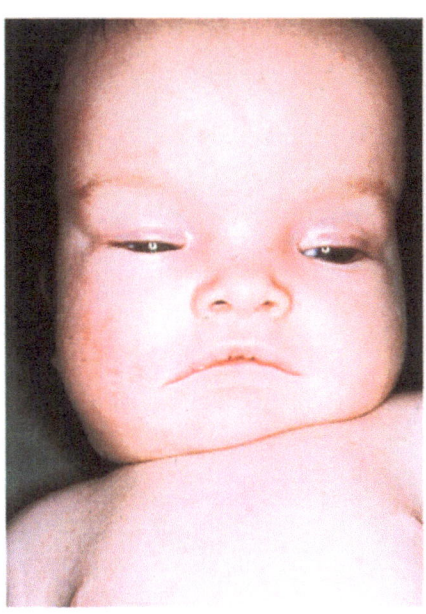

400 The forehead is large and there is a divergent squint

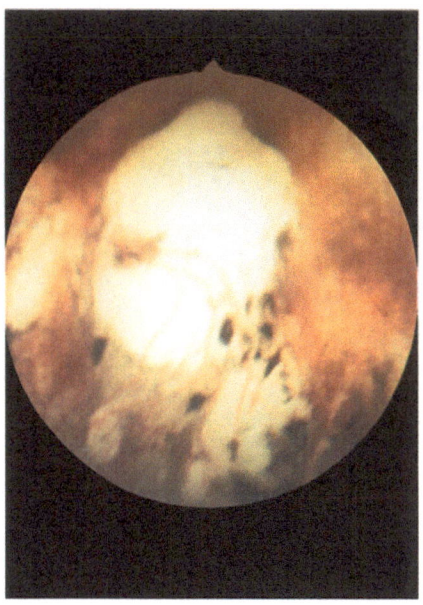

401 Retinal colobomas, especially in the Aicardi syndrome, look like holes and resemble toxoplasmosis which must be excluded by laboratory tests

The *Aicardi syndrome* (1969) or absence of the corpus callosum (ACC) with retinal colobomas and severe neurological dysruption in girls is still rarely diagnosed in the newborn period unless there is an affected sister. Reliable routine neurological examination of the newborn, however, will be alerted by unexpected neurological dysfunction maybe with a large head [399] and squint [400] before universal ultrasound arrives and has to whisper an embarrassing injunction to look for colobomas [401].

ACC itself varies enormously with regard to its apparent clinical significance. In one set of twins with severe hypertelorism [402, 403] both had ACC, yet in two severely handicapped boys of unremarkable facial appearance [404–406] low-priority CT scan revealed their ACC. In Patau's trisomy-13 and the holoprosencephaly sequence [cf. 370] ACC is almost incidental.

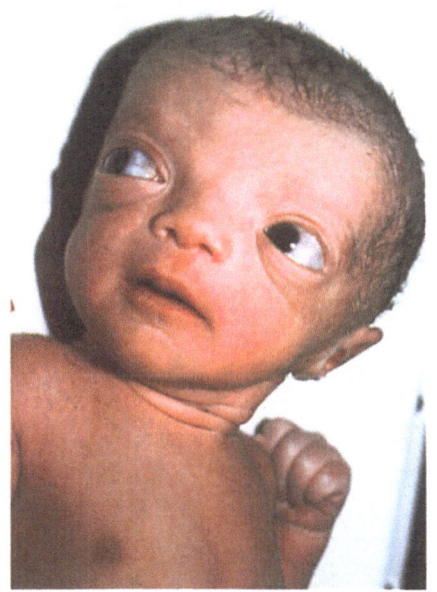

402

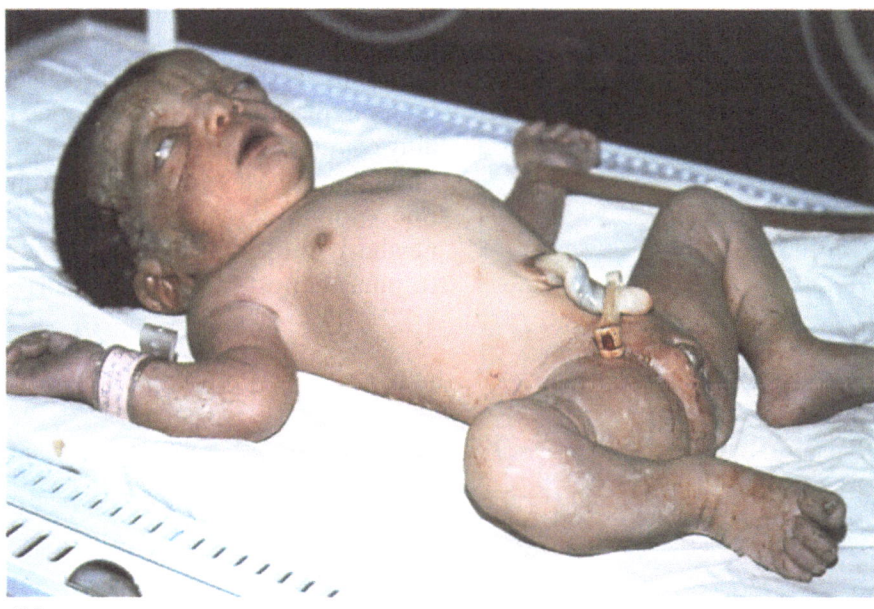

403

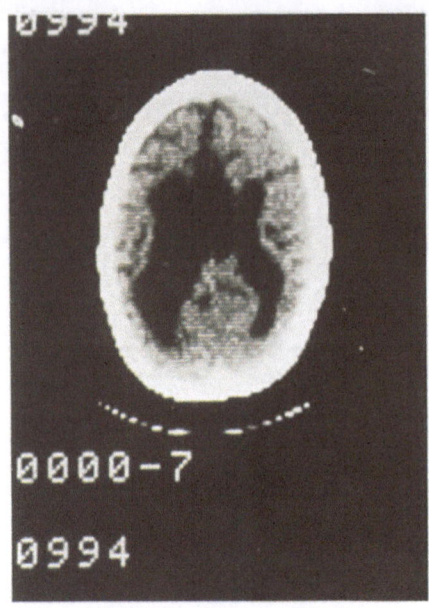

404 Child of a diabetic mother; this constitutes a risk

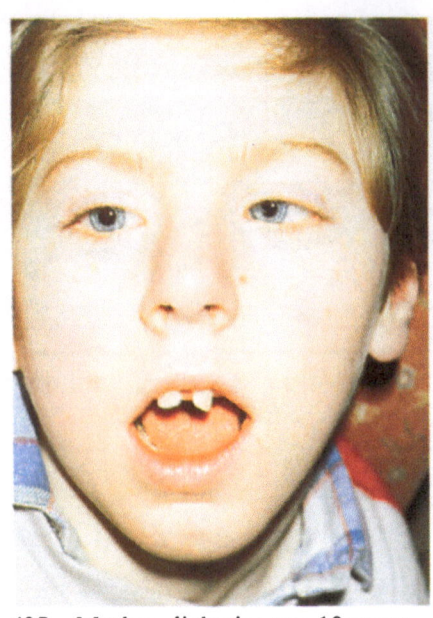

405 Mother diabetic; age 10 years

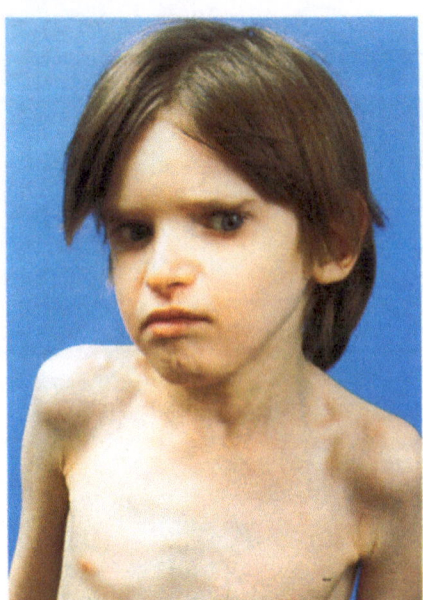

406 Age 12 years

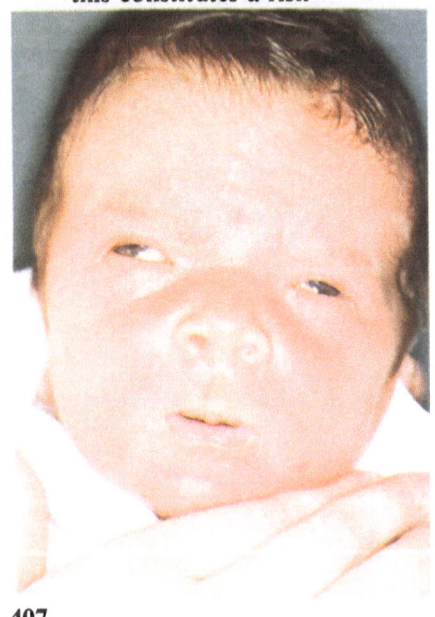

407

Sotos cerebral gigantism is rare but the facial appearance may be pathognomonic [**407**]: in addition to prominent hypertelorism there is squint with antimongoloid slant and prominent forehead. This macrosomic baby weighed 4.75 kg, the head circumference of 41 cm was disproportionately large and the ventricles were dilated. Another boy at 15 months [**408**] has cerebral gigantism (head 55 cm, height 92 cm, weight 13.5 kg) but facies dissimilar to the neonatal model.

Comment

These 'newer' facial dysruption syndromes were collected in one hospital over the past decade without a special search; very likely the number of examples is modest. Probably by accident there is diastasis between North America and continental Europe, but what of the black hole even for ascertainment in these islands, especially in this age of communication? It is not that the cases are not there: after a presentation of 10 cases of Opitz hypertelorism–hypospadias in Irish families to an audience probably connected with 25% of the paediatric units in these islands, a request on previous case recognition produced a show of 13 hands. This is just one condition readily recognized by competent primary care in the newborn nursery and where the results of delay cause psychosocial traumas almost incapable of correction.

408 Age 14 months

SURROUNDING TERRITORY MAY BE AFFECTED

Capillary naevi, so common that they are given the homely name 'stork marks', are most often seen on the upper lids [409] and forehead [410] or at the nape of the neck [411].

These marks are innocent and nearly always fade after some months, but in the nursery they represent a blemish and the mother requires a full explanation, in fact this is one of the items taking up most time in day-to-day nursery work properly performed.

An extensive florid mark may prove an exception to the rule: it is remembered as the hallmark of thalidomide embryopathy [412]. Such severe marks still command respect, they may point to serious trouble such as [413] the *Beckwith–Wiedemann* (EMG: *E*xomphalos, *M*acroglossia, *G*igantism) *syndrome*. The facial bones are hypoplastic, the eyes are usually prominent but here the impression is of mild hypotelorism. The immediate risk is of hypoglycaemia due to pancreatic islet hypertrophy (*gigantism*), surely an opportunity to prevent some of the mental handicap 'inherent' in this condition.

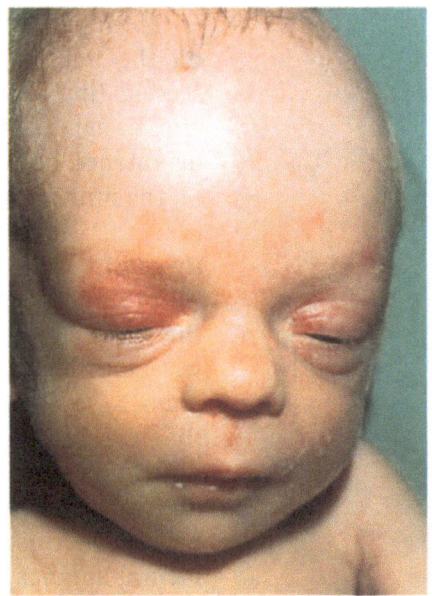

409 Now finding one of the nape of the neck impresses mother

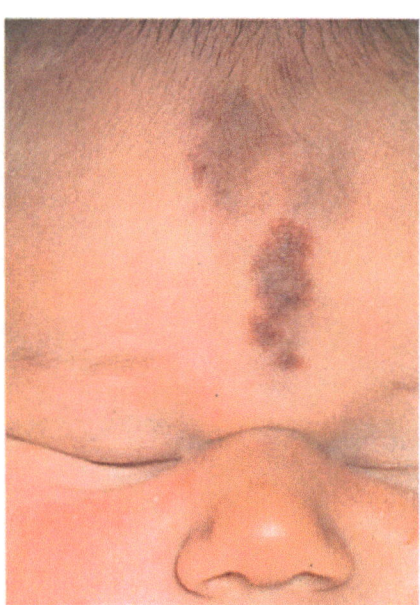

410

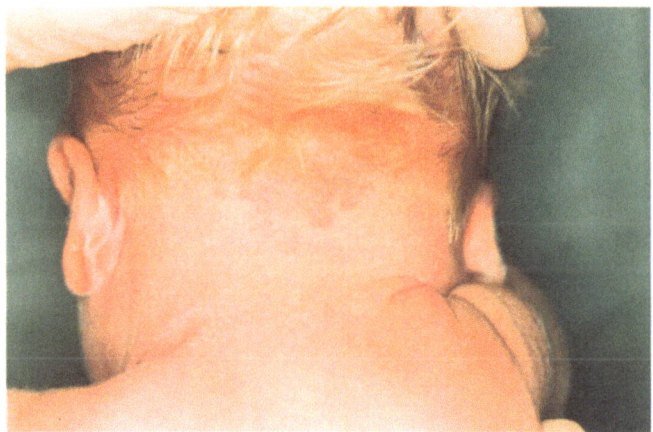

411 See!

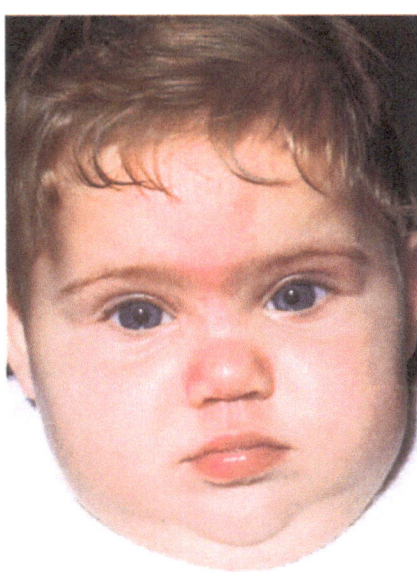

412 Also saddle nose

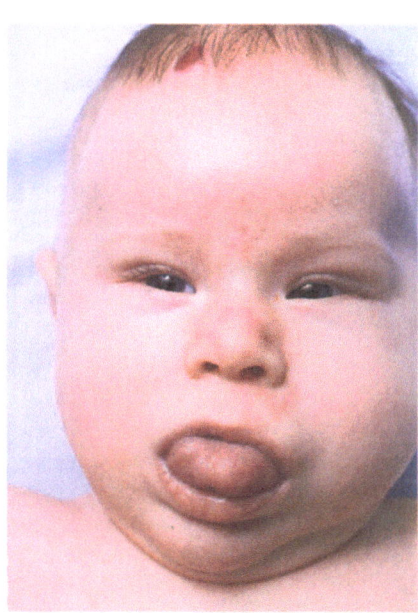

413 Hemihypertrophy

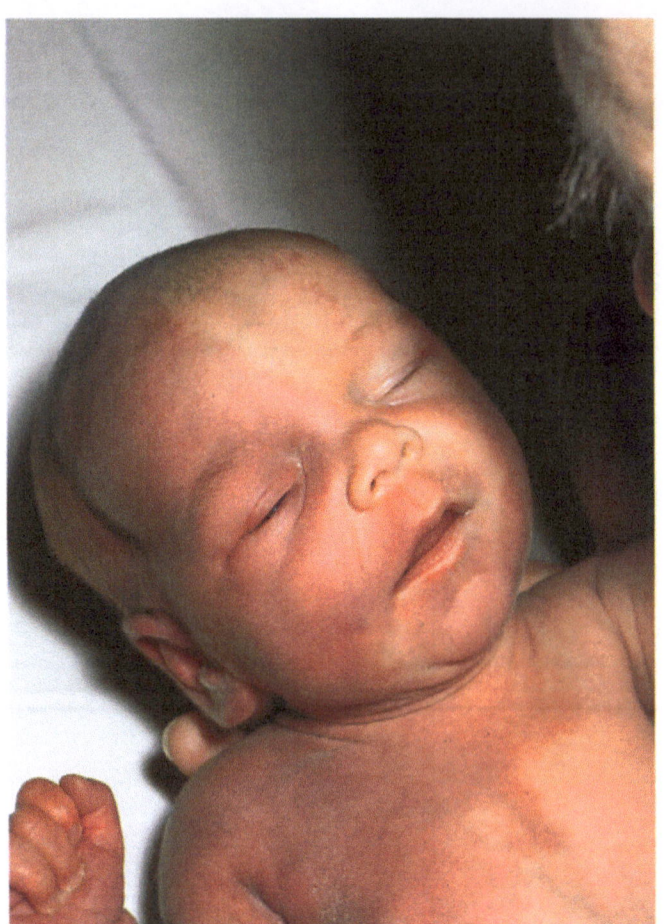

414 All trigeminal areas affected

Dense capillary naevi, 'port-wine stains' may be seen on the territory of the first (ophthalmic), and the second (maxillary), divisions [414] of the trigeminal cranial nerve. This is potentially serious, a probability heightened here by the association of extensive marks on the limbs, together with hypertrophy. The fear was that this could be *Sturge–Weber neuroectodermal dysplasia*, with lesions in the eye and brain as well. Before long the child developed *buphthalmos* [415], there was cloudy cornea with squint and epiphora. She was neurologically intact on clinical examination but a plain X-ray of skull showed the vault was smaller on the right side and the inner table thickened. All this was together taken to be diagnostic, then she collapsed under general anaesthesia. The prognosis is gloomy because there is a mark [416] on the brain, which causes mental handicap and fits; in due course the deposition of calcium and iron makes it opaque, and there is a 'tramline' pattern along the sulci. The uncontrolled fits and wild behaviour sometimes necessitate hemispherectomy [416]; the specimen on X-ray [417] shows the 'tramline' pattern fully.

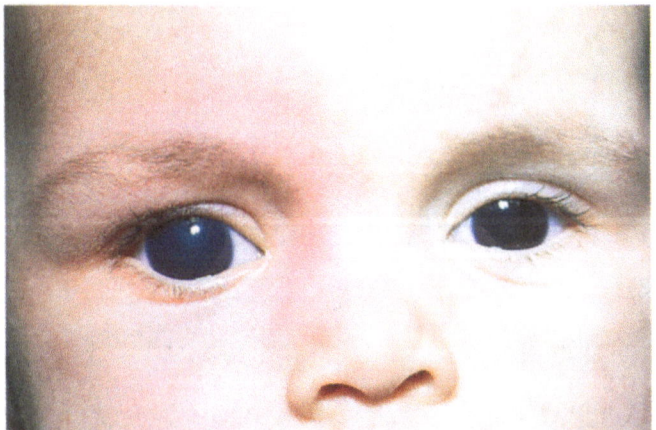

415 Clouded cornea

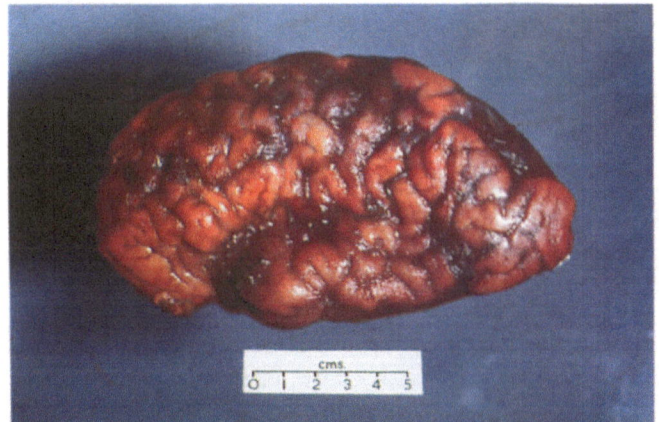

416 Hemispherectomy for wild behaviour

417 'Tramline' calcification and ferrugination

Another child with florid port-wine stains [418] and buphthalmos [419] who was alert and had had no fits has a normal CT scan after contrast injection; this excludes a vascular lesion of the brain surface. Happily, in the event *not* Sturge–Weber but certainly a 'damn close-run thing'.

Port-wine stains in one or other or even both [420] territories does *not* necessarily mean Sturge–Weber, but a dermatologist and neurologist or surgeon should be consulted and a cautious course pursued. This last child, seen at age 6 months, beautifully exemplifies the difference [421]; he is alert and neurologically intact, the birth mark has faded and shrunk, the only sign is a false impression of squint that is handsomely excluded by checking the corneal light reflections.

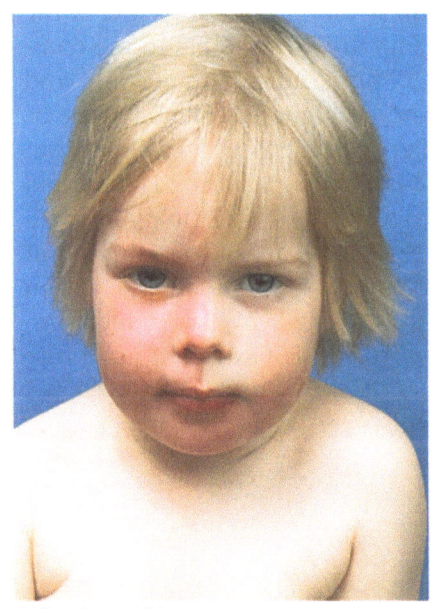

418　Age 3¾ years, a near miss. Glaucoma is almost unknown if the upper lid is spared

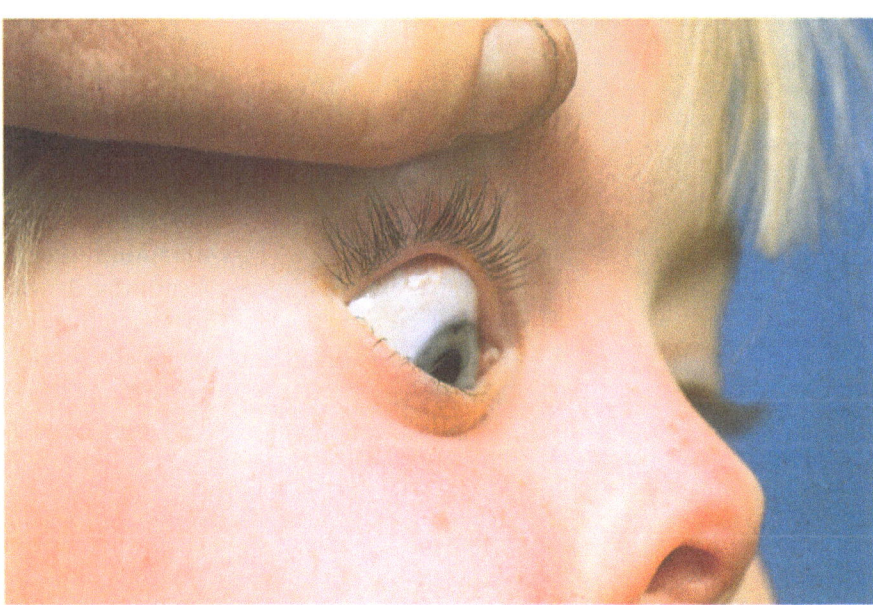

419　Oedema of globe after relieving trabeculectomy; scar of peripheral iridectomy in 12 o'clock position

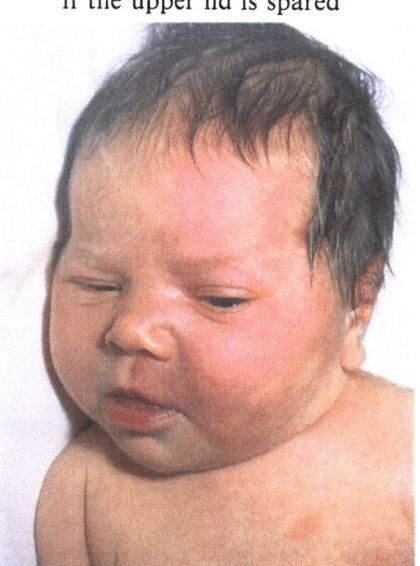

420　Dangerous marks . . .

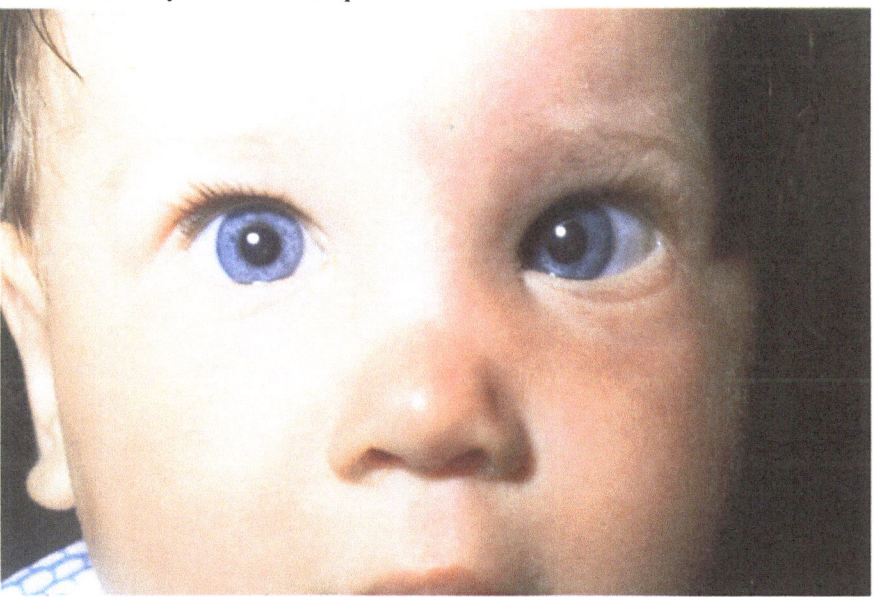

421　. . . But good early outcome

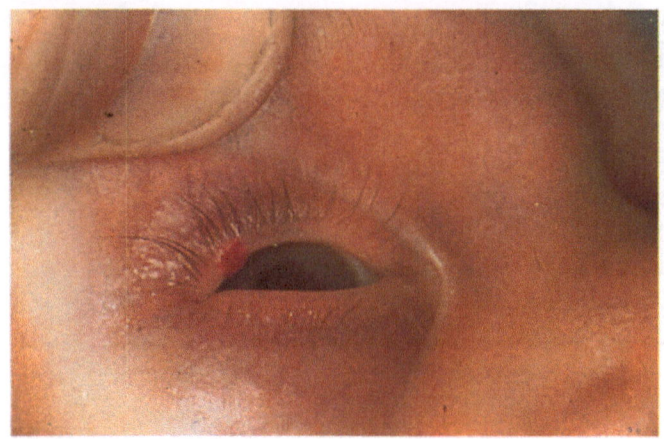

422

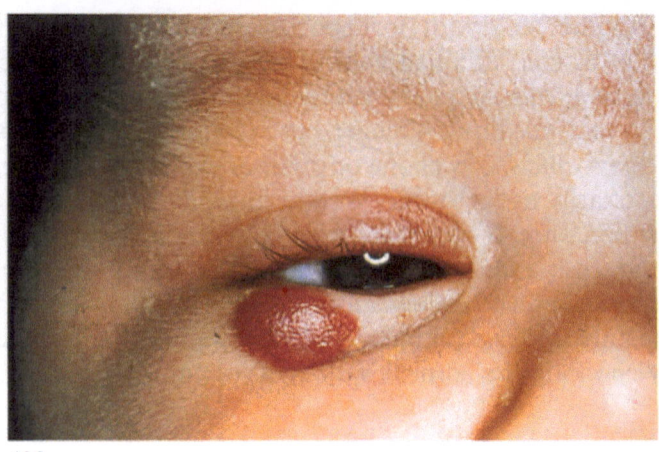

423

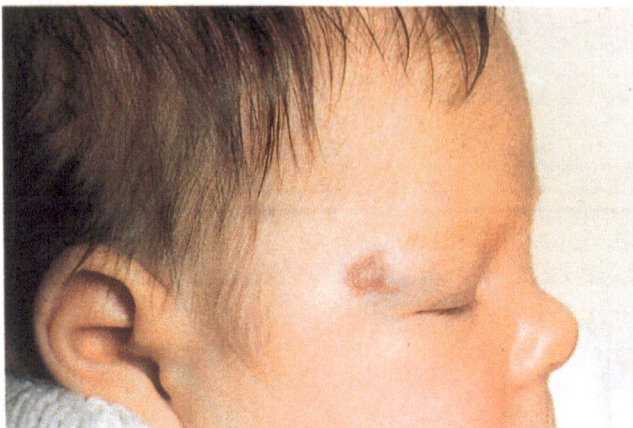

424

Cavernous haemangiomas may happen to be situated on the lids [422, 423] or close to the orbit [424]. Although 'birthmarks', not all are congenital, some appear only after a couple of weeks or so and complete spontaneous resolution in the pre-school years is the rule. This above all is an area irresistible to the compulsive therapist; when he is lucky enough to avoid early complications the outcome is brilliant, i.e., as good as the natural history of the untreated condition.

A good example is the extreme case a child unmarked at birth who began to develop a florid lesion [425] with maximum size and 'Fledermaus mask' distribution at 3 months. It was uncomplicated and thereafter began to fade; the residue at 4 years [426] had gone completely by school entry. At least 80% of these marks are gone by age 5.

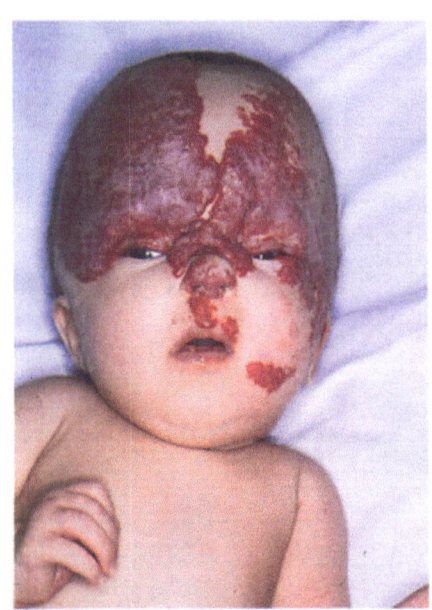

425   Age 3 months

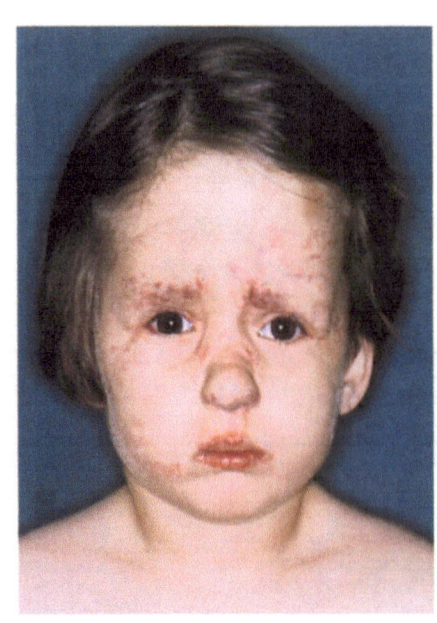

426   Age 4 years

A lesion of the upper lid must be watched with special care [427], since its growth may threaten amblyopia [428], one of the rare occasions when surgery is necessary. Malformation tends to be multiple, so when an apparently solitary lesion presents around the eye it is the rule that minute scrutiny all over [429] is essential, but it applies also closer to home [430], where something could remain hidden from casual search. When haemangiomas are multiple, [429], it raises the possibility of a generalized haemangiomatous disorder such as *Osler-Rendu-Weber*. During childhood the common problem is rectal bleeding, which should remind us to pay attention to that part of the gastrointestinal tract readily available for inspection [431]. In adult life the lesions are spider naevi ('hereditary telangiectasia') and then the common problem is troublesome epistaxis.

Another possibility, fortunately rare, is that vascular naevi near the eye could have generalized mesenchymal associations [432]. This child has the *Klippel-Trenaunay* disorder; she already shows some of the hypertrophy that may prove so troublesome [433] later on.

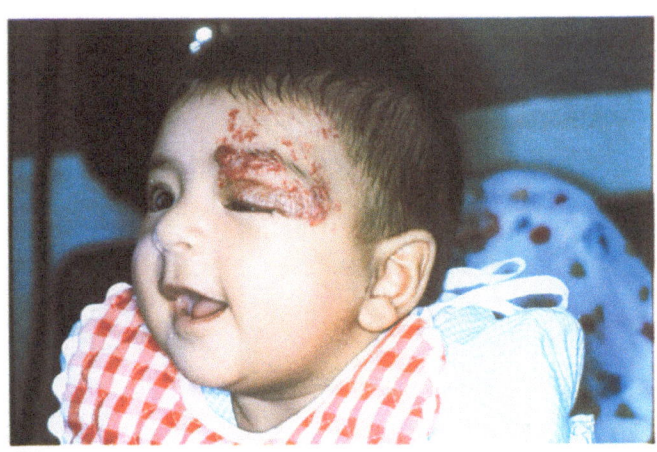

427

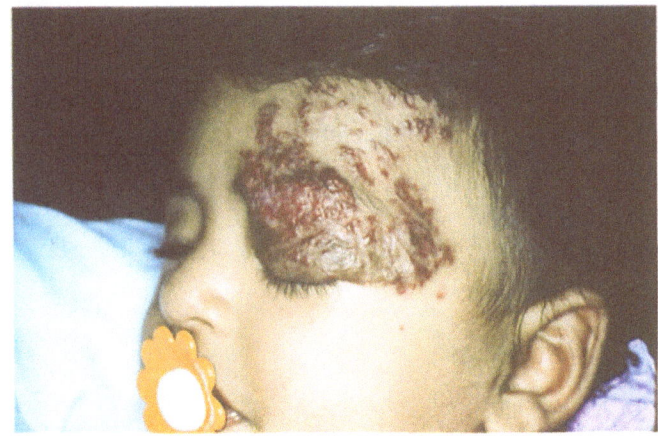

428

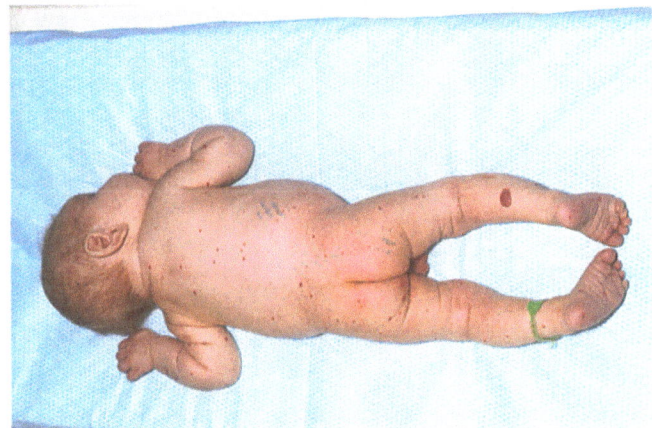

429 Age 3 weeks: lesions cropping freely

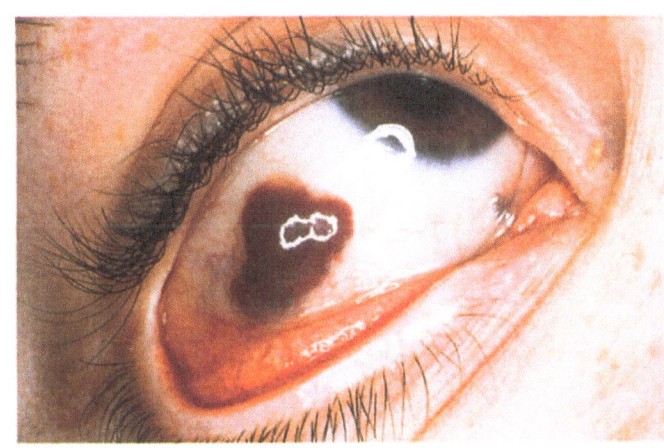

430

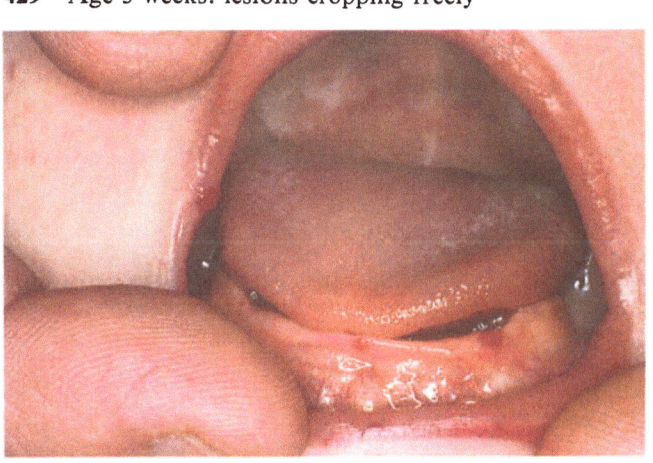

431

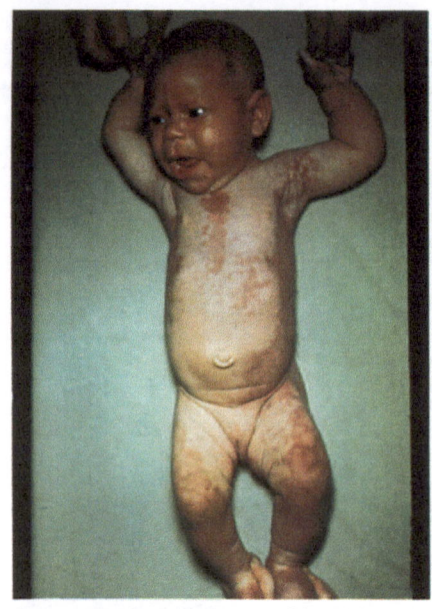

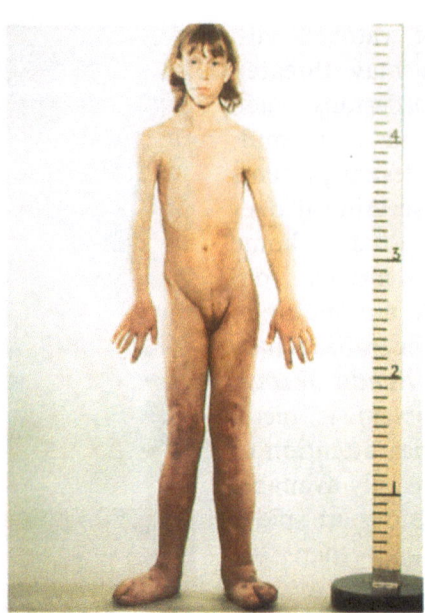

432   Age 1 month, considerable
       macrosomia

433

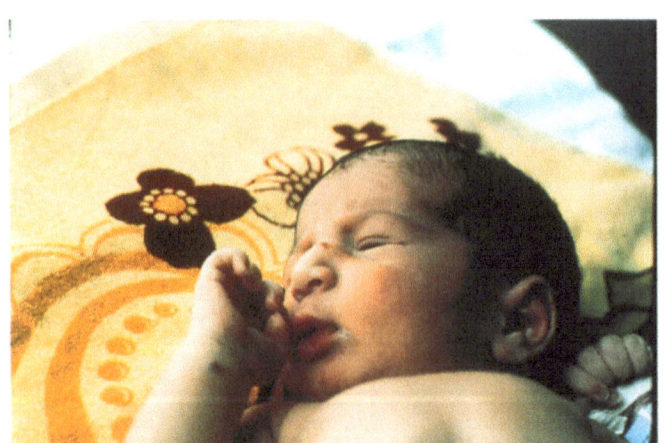

434   The lesion resembles a bilberry

An important lesson is learnt from a baby with a small presenting lesion [434] near the eye, at first associated with only two others. These were bladder-like and had a bluish bilberry tint; biopsy diagnosed the *blue rubber bleb naevus syndrome*. At its worst there is severe mental handicap with massive growth disorder [435, 436].

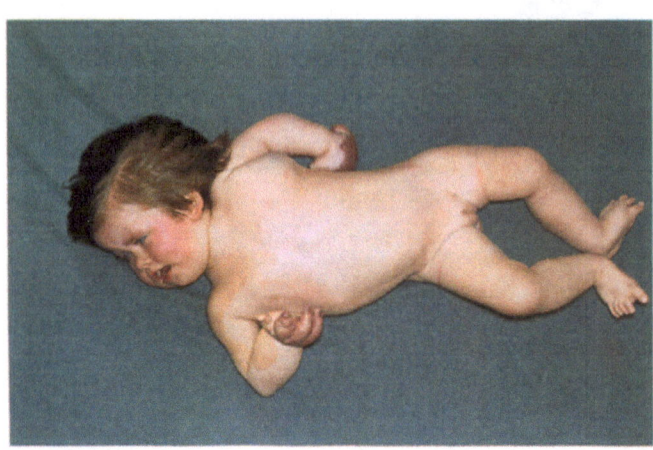

435

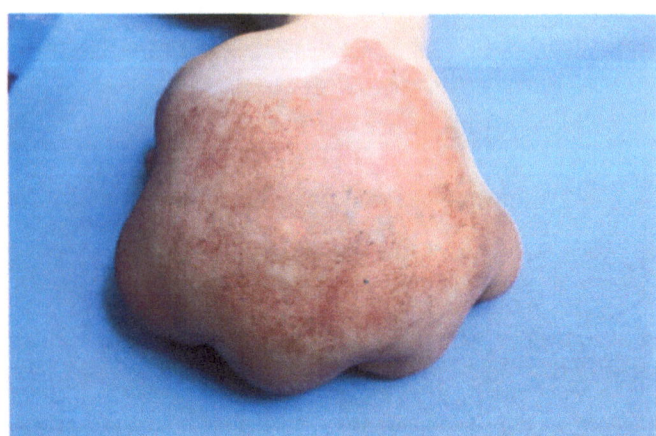

436

A pigmented mark on the lids, *cutaneous melanosis*, is most likely the *naevus of Ota* (the uveal tract and conjunctiva may be pigmented, *ocular melanosis*); its melanin at first shows blackish-blue [437, 438] through the skin. Later it is brown [439] and persists throughout life, and there is a slight risk of melanoma developing. This birthmark is commoner in Orientals; they too are liable to a similar mark on the shoulder, the *naevus of Ito*.

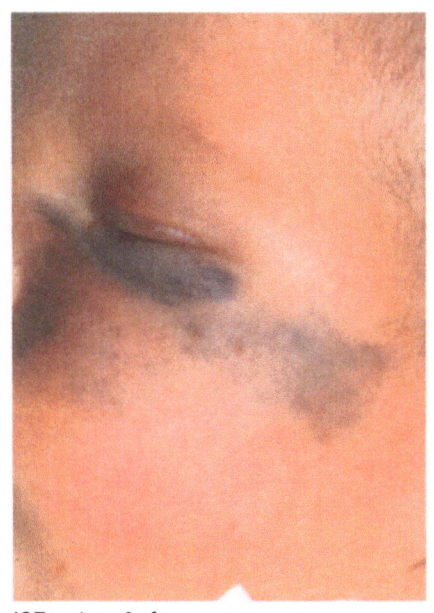

437 Age 3 days

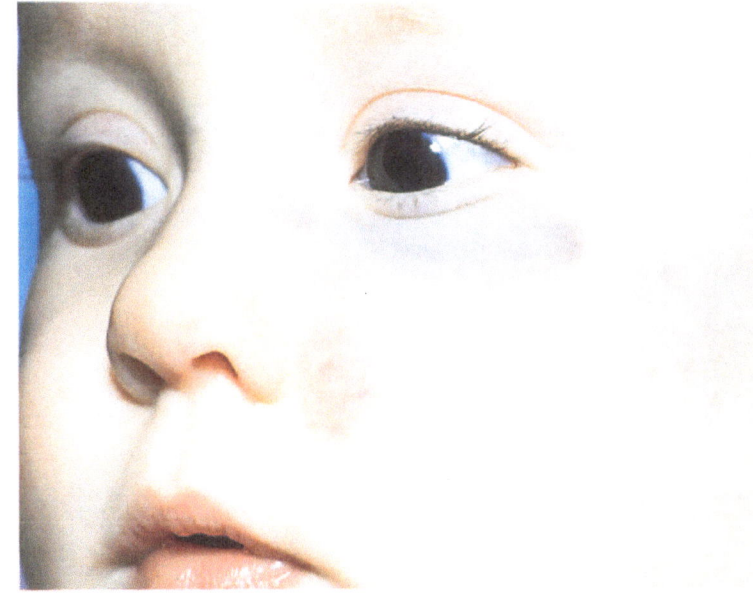

438 Age 9 months

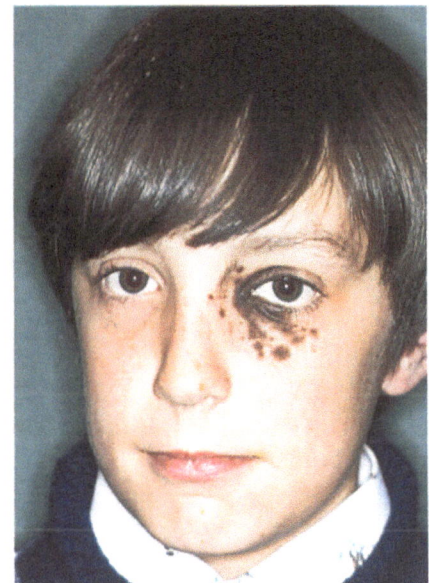

439 Age 12 years

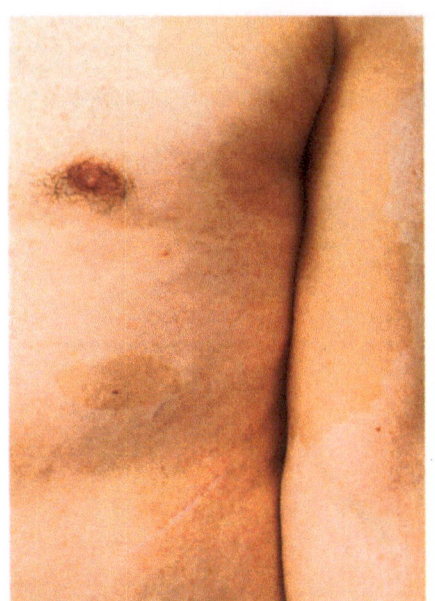

440 Von Recklinghausen

CONCLUSION

One might well look to the future with regard to finding two subtle neuroectodermal dysplasias, *neurofibromatosis* and *tuberous sclerosis*. We must first exclude:

(i) Cases forewarned by the family history [440–443].
(ii) Prenatal CT screening for periventricular opacities [448].
(iii) Cases seriously ill in the nursery [446, 447].
(iv) The expectation that an alert physician might find phakoma or a similar retinal lesion [449] by sheer clinical diligence.

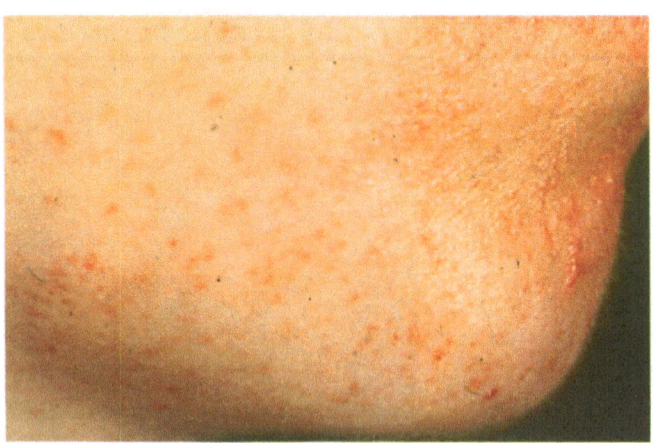

441 Adenoma sebaceum

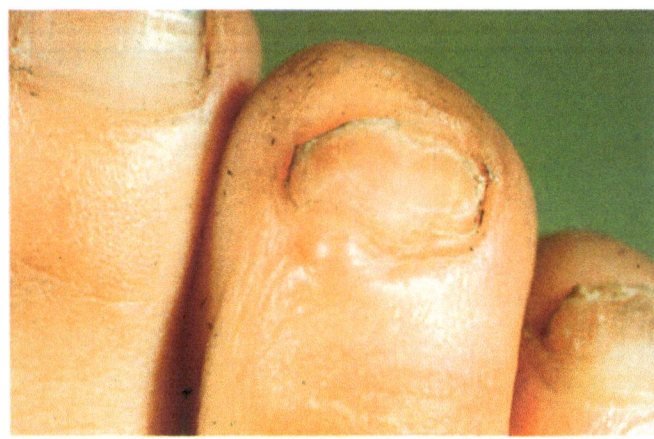

442 Periungual fibroma

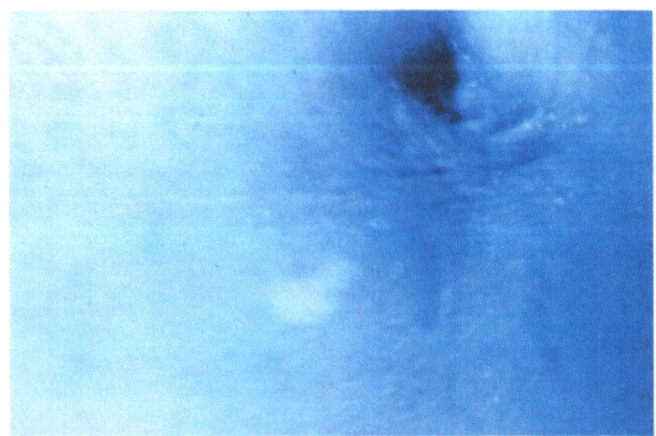

443 Achromic naevus in u.v. light

444 Café-au-lait spots

The practical challenge is to find neurofibromatosis (1/3000) or tuberous sclerosis (1/15 000 – 1/150 000) in the nursery. The answer is in the skin:

(i) Five or more café-au-lait spots [444] are strongly suggestive of neurofibromatosis.
(ii) Achromic naevi [445] suggest tuberous sclerosis very strongly; ultimately they are almost universal.
(iii) Adenoma sebaceum is rare in the nursery (3/59 in the Mayo Clinic series).

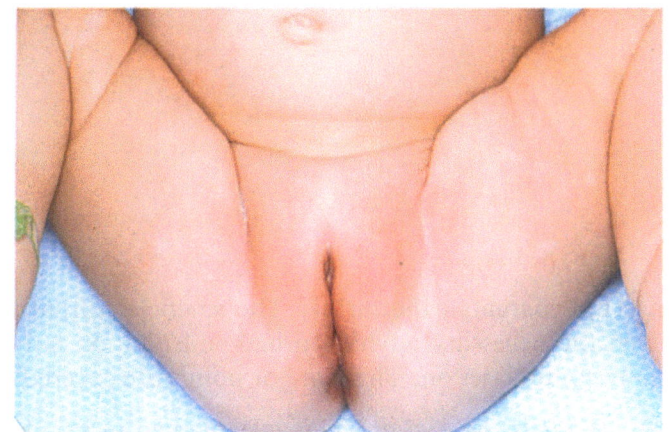

445 Achromic naevus left thigh

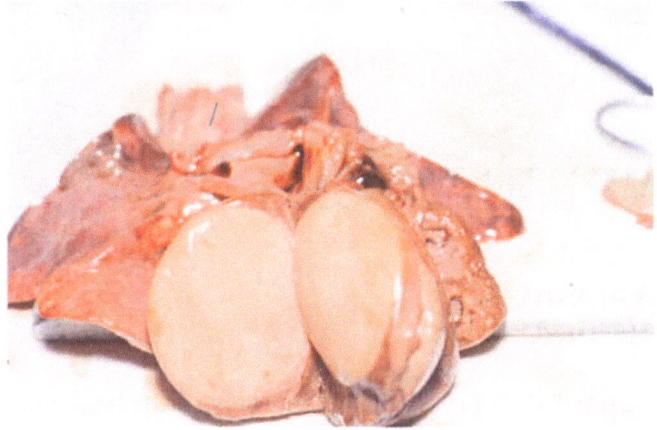

446 Rhabdomyoma of wall of heart

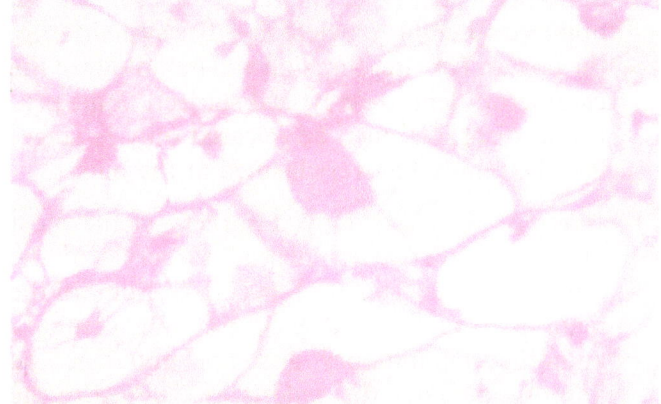

447 Pathognomonic 'spider cell' at centre

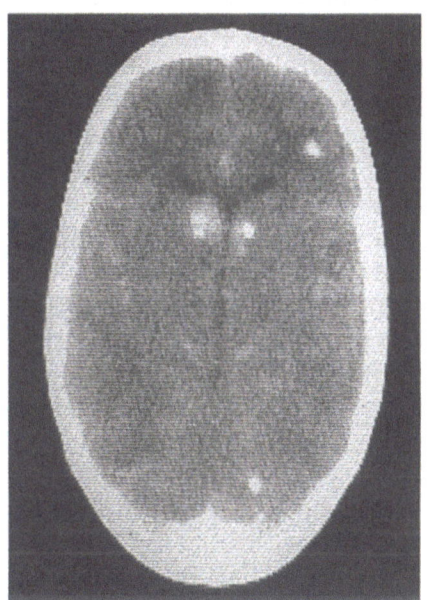

448 Typical 'candle guttering'

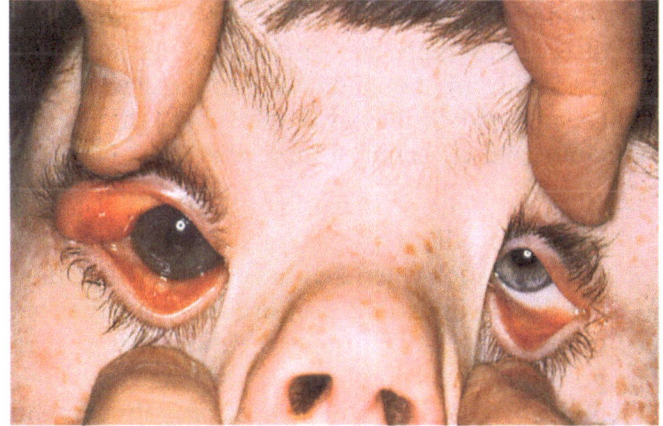

449 Von Recklinghausen

If we look at achromic naevi, can we shine UV light from a Wood's lamp on so many babies? The answer lies elsewhere and should not come as a great surprise:

'According to those parents who had been aware of the existence of the white spots before their attention was drawn to them by physicians, hypopigmented marks were first noted at birth or in the neonatal period.'*

The mother is usually right (again) and we have a new direct question: 'Have you noticed any coloured spots on the baby's skin, brown like a freckle or pale white maybe?'

*Hurwitz, S. and Braverman, I.M. (1970). *J.Pediatr.*, 77(4), 591

APPENDICES

APPENDIX I
THE DIAGNOSIS

The normal embryology and anatomy of the head and neck are more or less memorable for the average paediatrician but when the *pathological* dimension intrudes the going soon gets tough to the point where help is required. Even the perplexed should not send out a signal until the family history has been reviewed, the head-size measured personally, transillumination performed, neurological status including fundoscopy reliably determined, imaging done and the karyotype undertaken. Ocular abnormality always requires primary consultation by the ophthalmologist; the otorhinolaryngologist and plastic surgeon are next in demand, then any others as the local pathology dictates.

It is only in living memory that terms like 'cataract', 'coloboma',` 'hypertelorism', 'aniridia' or 'microphthalmos' (remember 'microcephaly'?) have come to be seen by paediatricians as 'generic' and not 'definitive' diagnostic statements; the accurate identification of sub-types is essential.

At the same time, for instance, the monolithic phenotype of Marfan has yielded homocystinuria, diet-responsive, likewise Crouzon has separated the milder Saethre–Chotzen, and similarly Treacher Collins the less serious Nager and Miller variants.

These forms of internal reclassification are matched by the development of embryopathic hazards in the environment, not least those that are iatrogenic, and possible exposure should always be kept in mind.

Finally, should one expose the experts to trivial stigmas in their special territories? This should be done wherever convenient; they will have useful observations to make and before long they will in this way make an early diagnosis of something important, and until then this modest diurnal rapport with the paediatrician, and the mother and baby together with the nurses and maybe an obstetrician, is an excellent and rewarding experience for all.

APPENDIX II
THE EXPLANATION

This, as we have seen, is the essence of the consultation. Ideally, the paediatrician and opthalmologist with any other necessary consultant (e.g. ENT, plastic surgeon) meet both parents in the nursery. The geneticist will have given the necessary advice, formal consultation normally comes later on. These major points are covered:

(1) *What is the matter?* This is explained in simple terms as far as is necessary at this time. The description tends to be more anatomical as opposed to embryological in other systems, e.g. the bowel. The site, function and pathology of the cataractous lens are a typical subject. Some profound disorders must be released only in stages lest the family be overwhelmed at the outset.

(2) *What is the plan?* Urgent surgery is the most important, thereafter interval surgery and the attentions of paramedical specialists. Some of the plan may be 'supervisory', e.g. Waardenburg audiology, mandatory and not mundane. In appropriate cases the child is ascertained to the Community Physician. With most alarming cases the specialist can reassure the parents that this child is not his worst affected child; before-and-after photographs may be shown at the outset and the family are soon inducted into the special clinic as soon as possible so the reality of the plan in depth and continuity is appreciated.

(3) *Why did it happen?* Curiously, this point has to be drawn out of the parents, quite often by a direct question when they have dried up, and then the doctor finds that they are surprisingly often under some wild misapprehension that he can promptly and completely dismiss and put their minds at ease. The gamut ranges from slippery elm through consanguinity to Roman Catholicism.

(4) *Could it happen again?* This is dealt with in Appendix IV, suffice to say here it is the least creditable part of medical management, whose guideline should be 'If you don't know, don't guess . . . find someone who knows'. The medical ignoramus is an optimist: 'never again, one in a million' (Down's syndrome), 'it should be all right if you have more children right away' (to Marfan father, not even Speedy Gonzales could outstrip the DNA). The lay ignoramus in the Mendelian minefield is by contrast a pessimist: 'all your children will have it' (facial clefting, hydrocephalus, exomphalos).

This aspect of the case should be discussed with the parents and any other responsible family member, e.g. grandparents if the parents are immature, informed siblings of Down's syndrome; the decisions and counselling are written in the case record and relayed to the family doctor and obstetrician. The local practice with regard to the registration of congenital abnormalities should be observed. Children proposed for adoption are a special important category. Nowadays, especially when the mother is unwed, the questions of paternity, consanguinity and incest are highly relevant and have come out of the cupboard, principally as far as the paediatrician, family doctor and paramedical staff of the maternity hospital and infant health centre are concerned.

APPENDIX III

bɼιseaɴɴ aɴ ᴅúᴄᴄas ᴄɼé śúιlιᴆ aɴ ċaιᴄ
Heredity shows in the cats eyes.

(Irish proverb)

GENETICS, SINGLE GENE EFFECTS HEREIN ILLUSTRATED, CRISP AND CLEAR-CUT*

Without any pretension to expertise or completeness this atlas is an ideal form of practical but useful presentation for the junior doctor in the nursery to learn and the tutor to use as an aid in teaching. Numbers written plain show that those illustrations demonstrate the mode of inheritance, while those in brackets indicate that only the proband is represented.

Autosomal dominant

Some cataracts 11, 12
Blepharophimosis 89–92
Some glaucoma 234, 235
Epicanthus 272
Osler–Rendu–Weber haemangiomatosis (429, 430)
Osteogenesis imperfecta, tardive 226, *severe* (225)
Saethre–Chotzen 305, 314, 315
Crouzon 315A, 315B
Apert (318), cf. Carpenter 319
Miller (328)
Nager (329)
Treacher Collins 327
Waardenburg 330–332
von Recklinghausen 249, 251, 210, 410–443
Oculodentodigital syndrome (335)

Probable autosomal dominant, or possibly X-linked, limited expression in female

Opitz hypertelorism–hyposapadias 375
Opitz–Frias (376)

Autosomal recessive

Galactosaemia (185)
Cystinosis (21, 98, 99)
Oculocutaneous albinism 197, 198, 199
Some ocular albinism 200
Caffey pseudo-Hurler GM1 gangliosidosis type I 169–173
Microcephaly, alaninuria 247
Riley–Day 289
Tay–Sachs, Sandhoff (168)
Numerous disorders featuring optic atrophy (166)
Opitz C trigonocephaly 385, 386
Carpenter syndrome (319)

X-linked dominant/autosomal dominant, lethal in affected male

Aicardi syndrome (165, 399, 400)
Oculofacial digital syndrome (OFD) type I (271)
Goltz (112)
Incontinentia pigmenti (70)

X-linked recessive

Hypohydrotic ectodermal dysplasia, 295–301
Fragile X syndrome, 196, the X chromosome is abnormal, there is a fragile site known to segregate with a mutant gene in X-linked Mendelian fashion.

Ocular albinism, some cases. Our patient (200) was a near miss, her sex precludes the diagnosis but one must show she is not Turner XO.

Aarskog syndrome may prove in time to be the commonest example, although no case was recorded it was easy to 'assemble' a replica (393–395) thanks to overlapping phenotypes.

Lowe's syndrome is not represented, in spite of *congenital* cataract, *congenital* glaucoma.

One will probably have to await the unravelling of family histories before the more obscure disorders are diagnosed in the neonatal period, for example Hunter (II) mucopolysaccharidosis, Fabry's sphingolipidosis, gyrate atrophy (hyperornithinaemia).

Sporadic (virtually certain)

Beckwith–Wiedemann 413
Goldenhar 349
Hemifacial microsomia 346, 347
Sotos 407

The Golden Rule

You can never say 'never' or 'always', which is to say there is no golden rule.

---

*One may well ask 'What of Robinow?', for instance. The simple answer in a word is 'heterogeneity'.

INDEX

References in **bold** type are to figure numbers.